COMPREHENSIVE GUIDE TO REMARRIAGE SUCCESS

Create a Strong Marital Base, Blend Families, Foster
Enduring Connections, and Shape a Shared Future

TAYLOR REED

Contents

Introduction

Who said lightning doesn't strike the same place twice? In love, I firmly believe it can—and does. Remarriage isn't just a rerun of your first go-around; it's a bold leap into the future, a testament to the unshakeable belief in the power of love and the human capacity for growth and change. This book isn't just another marriage guide; it's a lantern in the dark, guiding you through the unique journey of remarriage with empathy, practical wisdom, and a sprinkle of humor.

Now, let me hit you with a question that might feel a bit close to home: Is remarriage the ultimate test of hope over experience, or is it a grand declaration of our enduring belief in love? If you ask me, it's a bit of both. That hopeful voice inside us whispers, "This time, it'll be different. This time, it'll last."

My journey to writing this book started with a moment that could only be described as an epiphany during my second marriage. There I was, standing in the kitchen, realizing that while the ingredients (read: people) might be the same, the recipe for a successful remarriage needs its own unique spice mix. That moment, filled with laughter over a disastrously burnt dinner, was a turning point. It highlighted the universal craving for love, companionship, and the determination to make it work, no matter the obstacles.

Unlike other marriage manuals, this book dives deep into the nuts and bolts of remarriage. We're talking about the nitty-gritty details that make your second (or third, no judgment here!) marriage distinct. I've got you covered, from the importance of clear communication and financial planning to the joys and challenges of blending families and forging a new identity. It offers a comprehensive roadmap for navigating the complex terrain of remarriage with the latest research, expert advice, and real-life stories.

This guide is structured into four main parts—Laying the Foundations for Remarriage Success, The Dynamics of Blending Families, Building a Lasting and Fulfilling Relationship, and Cultivating a New Identity as a Couple—and is crafted to walk you through every step of the way. Whether you're contemplating retaking the plunge, already navigating the waters of a second marriage, or a professional supporting those on this journey, there's something here for you.

Approach this book with an open mind and heart, ready to explore remarriage's possibilities. It's about understanding that, while the path may have its share of obstacles, the destination—a relationship filled with love, understanding, and joy—is well within reach.

So, to you, the brave soul considering or embarking on this adventure, I offer a book and a companion. Together, we'll laugh at the quirks of merging lives (and last names), shed a tear over the challenges, and celebrate the victories, no matter how small.

Here's to finding happiness and fulfillment on your remarriage journey. Let's turn the page and start this adventure together.

ONE

Understanding the Journey Ahead

When you decide to give love another shot, the lessons you've learned from past relationships help guide the way. Getting remarried is a big decision, requiring looking inward and thinking things through. Relationships are complicated, so picking a partner for remarriage means understanding yourself well and being transparent about your shared goals and dreams.

Trusting Your Judgment in Partner Selection

When you think about getting remarried, your heart and mind are pulling you in different directions. But the best decisions happen when you balance what you feel and think. Understanding your past relationships can give you clues about what works and what doesn't, and research shows that being with someone who shares your values and life goals can make for a more satisfying relationship. Compatibility isn't just about liking the same things—it's about respecting each other, sharing interests, and having similar aspirations, and that's key for a successful remarriage.

Choosing a life partner means looking hard at your past, understanding what you need and learning from your experiences. It's not about dwelling on the past but using it to make smarter choices. Think of picking a partner like choosing a travel buddy: you want someone who can stick it out when things get tough, shares your sense of direction, and navigates what comes next. Emotional maturity, good communication skills, and similar life goals mark a partnership that's likely to last. Making these choices doesn't happen accidentally—it's about knowing what you need, want, and can't compromise on.

Asking yourself a few critical questions can help guide you: What have I learned from my previous relationships? What's important to me in a partner? Do my life goals align with those of my potential partner? These aren't just theoretical questions—they're practical tools to help you figure out what you need in a relationship.

However, it's essential to take your time. The excitement of a new start can make it tempting to rush into things, but it's vital to take the time to assess whether someone is suitable for you. Remembering the lessons from your past relationships can help you stay patient and choose a partner who matches and enhances your vision for the future.

Deciding to remarry is a big step. It's not just about finding love again; it's a hopeful and transformative choice that impacts your life. Choosing a partner for remarriage isn't just about following your heart—it's a thoughtful, creative process that blends your past experiences, current realities, and future hopes into a strong, fulfilling relationship. So, when you choose, ensure it's with your heart and head, aiming for a bright future together.

The Role of Self-Reflection Before Saying "I Do" Again

As we gear up for another trip down the aisle, looking at ourselves becomes more than just a routine check—it's a deep dive into what makes us tick. In this time of reflection, we listen to what our heart is saying, discovering what we truly want and need after everything we've been through. By doing this, we see how much we've grown, highlighting the significant changes since our last big relationship.

We grow and evolve with every experience, learning lessons and gaining wisdom. As we think about the future, it's about finding a deeper and better connection, not just going through the motions again. As you think about what you've learned about yourself, you start to see what you need in a partner this time—someone who wants to grow with you, not just fill a gap.

Getting remarried means you're all in—heart and soul. You must be honest about whether you're ready for this, covering all your bases—emotional, financial, and familial. It means dealing with any old baggage and genuinely understanding its impact. This emotional deep dive helps you start fresh. Since remarriage weaves together two lives and everything that comes with them, being financially prepared is just as important. And when families are joining together, it gets even more complicated, so you have to be ready for that, too.

You're not just finding another person to be with but choosing a life you want to build together. This vision for remarriage is about finding someone who resonates with your deepest self. When looking for a partner, it's more about who they are—their values, character, and dreams—than fitting some perfect image. Can you see a future where you both maintain your individuality yet share a common path? Do you feel like you're on the same wavelength?

A remarriage built on thorough self-reflection, growth, readiness, and a clear vision lays a strong foundation. Saying "I do" again means meeting each other in a place of deep understanding and mutual respect, not just proclaiming your love. It's about merging past experiences with future hopes to make a present filled with love, growth, and companionship.

Navigating the Emotional Landscape of Remarriage

Marriage is a ride with highs and lows, packed with memories that need a lot of thought and a deep understanding of its emotional layers. In this mix, emotional baggage from past relationships can linger, sometimes subtly, sometimes loudly. Addressing this head-on through honest reflection helps strengthen and purify your future relationship.

The first step is recognizing these emotional leftovers and understanding that they affect your feelings and reactions. Knowing them lessens their impact. You can deal with this baggage in many ways, whether through personal reflection or with help from a counselor who can offer unbiased, expert advice. It's not about wiping away these emotional marks—a part of your story—but making sure they don't overshadow a fresh start.

Being vulnerable in a new marriage is often seen as a weakness but a considerable strength. You must be open about your fears, anxieties, and deepest feelings. This kind of openness lets partners connect deeply, share concerns without judgment, and support each other without hesitation, laying the groundwork for a strong relationship where challenges are faced together, and vulnerabilities are supported.

However, the emotional side of remarriage isn't just about the couple; it also involves children from previous relationships. These changes can significantly impact them, and handling this with care is essential. Allowing kids to express their feelings about the new family arrangement and reassuring them that your love and support remain constant can help ease the transition. While this doesn't mean there won't be challenges, it does create a stable emotional foundation that helps kids adapt to their new situation.

The couple builds a foundation of shared emotional resilience by managing past emotional baggage, embracing vulnerability, and supporting each other and the kids through changes. This foundation, rich with mutual understanding, support, and open communication, sets the stage for their remarriage story. It's a narrative defined not by the absence of challenges but by the strength with which they are faced and overcome.

The Art of Starting Fresh While Honoring Your Past

Getting remarried involves balancing your past experiences with your current life. It's essential to appreciate your rich experiences while also making room for new successes in the future. As you navigate this balance, being aware and considerate is crucial. You bring memories of past love—complete with lessons, joys, and sorrows—while embracing the opportunities of a new relationship. The aim isn't to erase the past but to incorporate its lessons into your current life without letting it overshadow the new possibilities. This approach helps you value your history and be excited about your future.

Creating new traditions together is critical. They act as milestones in your journey, whether simple nightly routines, annual celebrations, or spontaneous acts of kindness. These traditions are the unique markers of your relationship, helping to establish your identity as a couple separate from your pasts. You create a bond based on mutual respect, love, and joy by consciously picking activities and celebrations that both partners enjoy. These new traditions then become the vibrant memories that fill your relationship.

Remembering past relationships is another crucial aspect. It means being able to talk about past experiences in a way that adds to, rather than takes away from, your current relationship. It's not about stirring up jealousy but about acknowledging how these experiences have shaped who you are. Open and sensitive conversations about the past can deepen trust and understanding between partners, showing how previous relationships have informed but not constrained your current choices.

Moreover, this thoughtful remembrance also involves how you handle your past internally. It's about giving space to your previous experiences in a way that honors their role in your growth without letting them overshadow your current happiness. This takes self-awareness and emotional maturity, allowing you to treasure the past while fully embracing the present opportunities.

In essence, starting a new chapter while honoring the past involves a continuous process of negotiation and adaptation. It requires patience, understanding, and a solid commitment to building a life that celebrates where you've been and where you're going. This balance provides the strength and resilience needed to nurture a relationship rich with the wisdom of the past and alive with future possibilities.

Communication: The Heartbeat of Remarriage

Communication is vital when two people come together to start a new chapter. It's all about chatting openly, understanding each other's gestures, and checking in emotionally regularly. Good communication goes beyond just trading information—it's about really connecting and making sure both partners feel listened to and valued.

Handling disagreements well means seeing them as chances to grow instead of just obstacles. Techniques like starting tough talks with kindness rather than criticism can help keep things calm. Regular "relationship check-ins" can also prevent minor issues from becoming big resentments.

Being open about what you need and want from each other is vital. It involves sharing your deepest desires and advocating for your well-being in the relationship. Clear, blame-free communication allows both partners to speak honestly without fear of judgment or back-lash, creating an environment where everyone feels supported and valued.

Listening well is equally important. It means paying attention and understanding the emotions behind the words. Showing you under-stand makes a big difference, whether by repeating what's been said or acknowledging the other person's feelings. It shows respect and helps build trust.

Communication is even more critical in remarriages, where baggage from past relationships might be present. It is the lifeline that helps navigate blending families, managing money, and sharing life goals. Challenges become opportunities for a stronger relationship when both partners commit to open, honest conversation.

Nonverbal cues like gestures and touch also play a significant role, offering support and love in ways words can't always express. A look or a touch can be all it takes to reinforce your connection.

Of course, communication isn't always accessible. Misunderstandings happen, words can be taken incorrectly, and emotions can get in the way. The key is staying committed to talking things out, listening with an open heart, and approaching each discussion as a chance to grow together. By seeing these moments as opportunities to strengthen their bond, couples can make their relationship even more solid over time.

In essence, communication is what keeps a remarriage strong. The constant effort to talk openly, listen actively, and respect each other builds a durable and loving bond. As both partners navigate the give-and-take of conversation, they find a shared rhythm that enriches their lives together.

Building a Strong Foundation With Premarital Counseling

Premarital counseling isn't just for first-timers—it's especially crucial for folks thinking about remarrying. It is vital for tackling potential issues and reinforcing the relationship's foundation. This deep dive helps build a partnership based on understanding, resilience, and joint growth.

Counseling starts by setting realistic expectations and helping couples handle the complexities of merging lives influenced by previous relationships. In a private setting, discussions aren't about dwelling on past relationships but understanding, accepting, and moving on. Couples get to shape their future together, recognizing past experiences but focusing on new beginnings. Counselors keep these conversations on track, ensuring expectations bring couples together instead of pulling them apart.

A big focus of premarital counseling is boosting communication skills. It's about more than just talking—it's learning to share emotions openly and honestly, which can clear misunderstandings. It turns potential conflicts into chances to connect more deeply because partners learn to tackle problems together, not against each other.

Blending families also gets a lot of attention. Counseling guides couples through the tricky aspects of bringing different family backgrounds together under one roof. It covers everything from setting boundaries to blending traditions, making sure new family bonds form smoothly and respectfully.

Through counseling, couples peel back the layers of their relationship to confront the raw truths that define them. It takes guts to face past failures and fears, but it sets a solid foundation for a strong marriage. Counselors are there every step of the way, helping build a marriage that's more than just a continuation of the past—a fresh start full of potential.

As the sessions go on, you'll see changes not just in how you communicate but in how you see your relationship. Misunderstandings become understanding, differences become shared goals, and the challenge of blending families becomes a chance to grow closer. This transformation starts a new chapter in your life, one filled with resilience, respect, and a solid commitment to make this partnership uniquely yours.

In short, premarital counseling for remarriage isn't just helpful—it's essential. It prepares you to deal with the intricacies of merging lives shaped by past relationships, setting you up for a union built on understanding, effective communication, and deep love.

The Significance of Financial Transparency

When you're getting remarried, being completely open about your finances isn't just an excellent idea—it's crucial for building trust and ensuring the relationship can handle whatever life throws. Sharing details about your financial past, debts, and future goals shows you're together and lays a strong foundation for your relationship.

Putting together a joint budget means more than deciding who pays for groceries; it's about mapping your future together. Sitting down to blend your finances shows you're ready to handle the ups and downs of life as a team. It's about more than just numbers; it's setting goals and chasing them together, with every dollar spent as part of a larger plan. The budget grows and changes with you, adapting to your life together.

Talking about debts you're bringing into the marriage requires guts and openness. Debt can weigh you down, but facing it together can strengthen your bond. By being upfront about what you owe, you're not just sharing a burden—you're turning it into a joint project. With a clear plan and shared goals, even paying off debt can feel like a victory you win together.

Planning your financial future means plotting a course that reflects your dreams and values. It's about more than just making it monthly; it's planning for retirement, investments, and savings in a way that supports both of your dreams. Financial advisors can be a big help here, steering you through the options and helping you make choices that keep your boat afloat through rough waters.

Ultimately, managing finances is about building a life together about more than just love. The practical decisions you make—from handling debts to planning your savings—tell the story of your partnership. Every discussion at your kitchen table, every plan made during late-night talks, adds to this story, crafting a future built not just on romance but on a shared commitment to making your lives work together.

Legal Considerations Before You Remarry

Getting remarried adds many legal issues to the mix, which are essential to resolve for both partners and their families. Understanding the legal side of things is crucial to protecting everyone involved.

Prenuptial agreements are a big part of this. They used to get a bad rap, but now they're seen as an intelligent move. These agreements help couples lay out the financial details of their marriage, like who owns what and how debts and assets should be handled. Far from being a sign of mistrust, a solid prenup shows that both people are into being open and fair from the start. It heads off potential money arguments and sets clear expectations. When making a prenup, it's vital to have open chats about each person's financial past and hopes for the future. Lawyers specializing in family law can help tailor these agreements to the couple's situation.

Estate planning also becomes super crucial in remarriages. It's not just paperwork—it's about making sure your stuff goes where you want it to after you're gone, like ensuring kids from a previous marriage are taken care of while respecting the new relationship. This part often involves tough conversations and careful balancing to ensure everyone's treated fairly.

If there are kids involved, remarriage can shake up existing custody and child support arrangements. Sometimes, you need to go back to the lawyer to update things. It's about finding a balance that respects the kids' needs and the rights of all parents involved.

By sorting out these legal issues—like prenups, estate plans, and custody—couples set themselves up for an emotionally and spiritually fulfilling and legally solid relationship. It's about facing tough topics head-on and strengthening trust and respect. This legal readiness shows commitment to each other and to blending families smoothly.

These legal steps aren't just formalities; they're about protecting and expressing care for each other. They help ensure that the new marriage can handle future challenges well. Tackling the legal aspects of remarriage is part of building a solid foundation for a future that's as legally secure as rich in love and partnership.

Aligning Your Spiritual and Ethical Beliefs as a Couple

Syncing up your spiritual and ethical beliefs can strengthen your connection when you remarry. It's about finding common ground in your deepest values and beliefs, which helps solidify your bond for the long haul.

If you're from a different spiritual background, the key is to be curious, not aggressive. It takes a lot of empathy and a commitment to understand each other to make an interfaith relationship work smoothly. You've got to dig into conversations beyond differences, finding shared values that go deeper than any specific religious doctrines. These discussions, if you keep an open mind and heart, can reveal a set of shared ethics that guides your decisions and actions, setting a solid base for your life together.

Sharing and respecting each other's spiritual traditions isn't just educational; it deepens your emotional and spiritual connection, lasting your whole life together. It's not about compromising your beliefs but expanding your understanding and appreciation of your partner's. This journey helps you both create a unique spiritual path that respects your traditions while celebrating what you believe together.

Couples who agree on these core values build their marriage on a solid foundation of respect, honesty, and integrity. Honest and open communication creates a safe space that strengthens trust. This trust is crucial in dealing with differences and challenges, especially when blending families and lives in a remarriage.

Connecting to a faith or spiritual community can also be a huge help. These groups offer support and wisdom that can guide you through the ups and downs of marriage. Getting involved can deepen your connection to shared values and others living by similar principles.

Participating in community activities can enrich your relationship in many ways. It ties your journey to a larger story of faith and ethics, and mentors from these communities can offer valuable guidance. Plus, involvement in service or activism projects can strengthen your commitment to living out your values together.

Ultimately, when you remarry, it is more than just joining your life; it's a chance for exploration and growth. It's about listening to each other, challenging your assumptions, and embracing the diversity of spiritual and ethical beliefs. By aligning your beliefs and values, you build a strong base for your relationship and find joy in your shared journey toward deeper understanding, respect, and love.

Setting Realistic Expectations for Remarriage

To make a remarriage work, you've got to be flexible and ready to handle everything that comes with it—like blending families, sorting out money issues, and merging different life paths. It's about being open to change and adjusting to each other so you can grow as individuals and as a couple. Being adaptable helps strengthen your relationship.

The first thing to do is to bust some common myths about remarriage. There's this misleading idea that when you remarry, it will fix everything from your past, and only happy times await. While it's a nice thought, it needs to be more accurate. Every relationship, even a remarriage, comes with its own set of challenges. Facing these challenges head-on allows couples to set realistic expectations and accept that building a life after divorce or losing a partner is complex. It's not about cutting down on the excitement; it's about having a balanced understanding of marriage that appreciates the good times and prepares for the tough ones.

Flexibility is critical because life is constantly changing. Remarriage can bring many challenges, like bringing together different families, figuring out finances, and aligning your life goals with someone else's. Your relationship needs to do more than just tolerate change—it must embrace it. Couples who adjust well to each other find their unique way forward, letting them grow individually and together. Overcoming challenges along the way only strengthens your bond.

It's also important to celebrate your differences. While people often talk about how vital compatibility is, your differences can make your relationship richer. Seeing things from your partner's perspective can turn potential conflicts into chances for understanding and growth. Living together teaches you how to compromise, negotiate, and respect each other, which are all crucial skills in any marriage.

Setting realistic expectations is like carefully building a plan for your life together, considering life's good and the challenging parts. This plan should reflect a hopeful look at the future without ignoring the lessons from the past. You've got to be cautious yet bold as you balance your optimism with the wisdom you've gained from previous experiences.

On this journey, keeping it real doesn't mean you can't have romance or passion. These elements naturally mix into a relationship grounded in reality but still aim high. Realistic expectations help guide you through remarriage, anchored by your deepest values and shared dreams. True love shows itself in big romantic gestures and everyday ways you understand, compromise, and support each other.

TWO

Healing and Growing from Past Relationships

T hink about the end of winter when you can see what's left from last season alongside the new growth. This mix of old and new is similar to bringing past relationship experiences into a new marriage. It's essential to be aware of these past influences and manage them carefully so that they contribute positively to the new relationship.

Understanding the Shadow of Past Relationships

Past relationships can influence how you act and feel in a new marriage. For example, you might find yourself arguing over something trivial, like weekend plans, but the real issue might be unresolved feelings from the past. It's important to recognize these emotional triggers—small things that upset you more than they should because they remind you of past issues.

Discussing what bothers you in a supportive environment where you don't feel judged is crucial to preventing past hurts from affecting your current relationship. When you and your partner can openly share your concerns and work through them together, you're better prepared to deal with similar issues in the future.

Being aware of your own emotions is essential. You must explore your feelings to understand how your past relationships impact your current ones. This might involve journaling, meditating, or even therapy. A clear view of your emotional state helps prevent old problems from disrupting your new relationship.

This type of self-awareness isn't just about solving problems; it's also about healing and growing from your experiences. It makes your new marriage a fresh start, allowing you to build something extraordinary without the weight of old baggage.

Textual Element: Reflection Section

- **Reflect on a recent disagreement or emotional reaction within your relationship.** Can you trace this reaction to a specific experience or pattern in a past relationship? Write about this connection and consider discussing your insights with your partner.
- **List potential emotional triggers that you've identified in yourself and your partner.** Discuss strategies for managing these triggers together, emphasizing empathy, understanding, and support.

This section is about helping you and your partner determine how your past relationships might affect your current relationship. By thinking about this together, you'll understand each other better, setting you up for a relationship built on respect, support, and growth.

It's essential to recognize the influence of your past relationships without getting stuck on them, which requires patience, empathy, and a real commitment to growing together. Think of it as nurturing a garden—it's all about using your past experiences to enrich what you're growing, setting you both up for a great future together.

The Process of Forgiveness: Letting Go of Old Hurts

Forgiveness isn't just about healing and feeling better—it's also a huge part of getting ready for a new marriage. It's way more than just saying "it's okay." It takes a lot of guts and deep character to forgive. When you forgive, you relinquish old grudges that tie you to past hurts, freeing you to open your heart again and let new love in.

Forgiving Yourself

Starting to forgive yourself involves some honest soul-searching. It's difficult to admit your mistakes and weaknesses from past relationships. But learning to forgive yourself is a big step toward healing. Everyone makes mistakes—it's part of being human. The key is learning from these mistakes rather than beating yourself up.

You might start by thinking about times in your past relationships when you weren't your best self or hurt someone without meaning to. The point isn't to feel bad about yourself; it's to understand and accept these moments so you can move on. Writing forgiveness letters to yourself can be a constructive way to deal with these feelings. It's about affirming that you deserve happiness and love despite your past.

Forgiving Others

Forgiving your ex is a big step that doesn't need them to apologize. It's about letting go so you're not feeling bitter, which can ruin your happiness and new relationships.

It all starts with admitting you're hurt. It's okay to feel and acknowledge those emotions. Then, try to see the big picture of your past relationship—think about the misunderstandings and all the personal stuff you may have been dealing with that contributed to the split. It's not about excusing anyone's bad behavior but about seeing things from a human perspective, making forgiving easier.

For some, forgiveness might mean having a final talk with their ex to get closure or just expressing all those pent-up feelings. For others, it means quietly letting go of the pain and moving on. Either way, forgiving means giving yourself the freedom to live fully and love again.

Letting Go

Forgiving yourself and others and finally letting go is all about choosing not to let old hurts weigh you down anymore. It's the most challenging part because you must move past the old stories you've told yourself about love and relationships.

If you're ready to let go, it's all about shifting your focus from the past to the future. Staying in the moment and looking forward helps. Sometimes, doing something symbolic like writing down your grudges and burning them can feel free. Picking up a new hobby or routine can also help you move forward, giving you a fresh sense of who you are outside of your past relationships.

When you get remarried, it's a shared journey of letting go where both of you support each other. It means creating a space to share your vulnerabilities—not as burdens but as ways to connect more deeply. The relationship strengthens when both partners can forgive and move past old pains.

Forgiving yourself, forgiving others, and letting go is crucial to building a healthy, understanding, open-hearted remarriage. Love at its best is about embracing each other and letting go of the past. It's tough, but this forgiveness journey can lead to a remarriage full of love, understanding, and new beginnings.

Learning from Past Mistakes: Growth Mindset in Action

Turning your past mistakes into lessons is all about changing your perspective. It's not about beating yourself up; it's about evolving. You can work toward a healthy and lasting remarriage with a growth mindset. This process helps you build better relationships instead of getting stuck in regret.

It starts with recognizing the patterns that caused problems in your previous relationships. You used to shut down instead of discussing conflicts, which led to more misunderstandings and distance. It's challenging, but you need to be honest about these habits. It's not about beating yourself up; it's about understanding what went wrong and breaking these cycles.

The real work focuses on personal growth, not just taking up new hobbies. It means developing better emotional awareness, empathy, and resilience. Practices like mindfulness can help you become more tuned into your thoughts and feelings, making navigating your emotions much easier. You can also expand your mind by taking courses or participating in creative projects. Growing like this doesn't just change you; it improves your relationships.

This process is about seeing life's challenges as chances to learn and grow, not threats. It's about making active choices that reflect what matters to you. For someone heading into remarriage, this might mean being more open about what you need and setting boundaries that respect your self-worth.

Embracing a growth mindset is about learning from your past and being open to change. Sure, it can be challenging. You might doubt yourself or slip back into old ways. But these moments show how resilient and committed you are to making things work this time.

Lessons from the past shouldn't trap you; they should empower you. They're not marks of failure but proof that you've grown. With this approach, remarriage isn't just a repeat of the past; it's a fresh start. It's a chance to build a relationship based on mutual respect, understanding, and love fueled by the wisdom you've gained.

In short, the journey to a successful remarriage, driven by personal growth, shows how much you can transform. It turns past relationships from regrets into stepping stones for a future where love is richer and more informed by experience.

The Importance of Closure: Saying Goodbye to What Was

Closing the chapter on past relationships is more than just turning a page; it's about making peace with your history so you can fully dive into a new marriage with an open heart. It's not just about forgetting the past; it's about settling things in a way that frees you up for what's next.

Depending on your situation, there are a few ways to find closure. A straightforward chat with your ex can clear the air and tie up loose ends if you're on good terms. This kind of talk can be challenging—it means facing up to old hurts—but getting through it can lighten your emotional load.

Another way to mark the end of an old chapter and the start of a new one is through a personal ritual. This could be like letting go of old keepsakes or writing a letter you never sent. These rituals can help you honor the past while making way for the future, and they can be powerful, especially if you share the moment with close friends or family.

A big part of moving on is reflecting on what you've been through—thinking about the good, the bad, and how you've grown. This might mean some quiet time to think, write in a journal, or discuss things with a therapist. Understanding and accepting your journey can help ease you into being ready for a new relationship.

Ensuring your heart is in it is crucial when getting ready to remarry. That means looking honestly at how past relationships have shaped you. You want to ensure you bring the best of your past, not letting it hold you back.

Closure isn't just an ending; it's setting the stage for a fresh start. When you're ready to move on, you're not just free of past hang-ups —you're poised to embrace a new partnership with all the wisdom you've gained. It's about acknowledging your past and using it to enrich your future.

So, as you step into a new marriage, see it as a chance to bring everything you've learned about love, yourself, and life. Closure lets you start this next adventure unburdened and open to all the possibilities of a partnership built on a clear, strong foundation.

Embracing Your Story: The Power of Your Personal Journey

Our experiences, good or bad, win or losses shape us. As we step into remarriage, we must embrace every part of our story—every line, chapter, and word. It's not just about recognizing who we are but fully accepting ourselves. There's real power in owning and using our story to connect more authentically and deeply.

Part of embracing who we are involves treating every experience with respect, whether it's a win that boosted us or a setback that brought us down. It takes guts to look at your story and see each stumble and success as valuable lessons. Past relationships and marriages become key parts of our narrative, not just remnants of our past. They aren't stains on our record; they're proof of our commitment to living fully, to seeking connection, love, and understanding.

When we share our life story with our partner, it's more than just recounting events. We're opening up about the emotional paths we've walked, the dreams we've held onto, and the scars we carry. This sharing should be a safe space where neither of you feels judged. It's about honoring each other's past, learning from it, and using that knowledge to deepen your connection. True intimacy grows from this fertile ground of shared truths, where conversations are heartfelt and profound.

Our resilience, born from our experiences, is crucial. It's not just about getting through tough times; it's a testament to our unwavering desire to find happiness and meaning, no matter what life throws our way. Recognizing and celebrating this resilience shows that we can handle life's challenges together and are ready for all the new union's possibilities. It creates a relationship based on mutual respect and shared strength, where you face challenges together, confident that you can weather any storm.

So, embracing our whole story isn't just about making peace with the past; it's about weaving these experiences into the foundation of a new marriage. In this new chapter, your past doesn't overshadow your present; it lights the way to a future filled with hope and new possibilities.

By fully accepting our past and sharing it openly, remarriage becomes more than just a second chance—it's a celebration of what's been and a hopeful look at what can be. It's an opportunity to build something genuine and strong, a relationship that honors your journey and the endless possibilities ahead.

Healing Together: Supporting Each Other's Past Wounds

Healing together is a big part of making a remarriage work. Working through past issues as a team builds a strong, healthy bond that can last long. This process is all about growing empathy, trust, and a deep connection with each other so you can build a lasting marriage.

Empathy is enormous here. Empathy grows when you share stories about your past hurts and challenging times and listen to each other without judgment. Being fully present and tuning in when your partner opens up about their scars shows them they're safe to be vulnerable. This kind of empathic listening means that even the tough stuff gets treated with kindness and understanding.

One practical way to show you're both committed to healing is to engage in healing activities together. Attending therapy to work through personal issues or conflicts between you can be a solid way to come together. Therapy with a professional who specializes in emotional healing can help you both address your past, understand your present, and prepare for a future without trauma. Couple retreats that focus on healing and connecting are also beneficial because they offer a supportive environment to engage in the healing process away from daily distractions. These experiences can strengthen your bond and deepen your trust in each other.

Trust is the real deal in relationships, and it gets even stronger when you're healing together. Seeing how committed your partner is to working through their stuff and helping you with yours builds a deep trust. Every shared emotional moment, every vulnerability shown, and every step taken together towards getting better solidifies this trust. It turns your relationship into a safe space where both of you know you can count on each other through the good and bad times. This solid, trust-filled foundation will support your future together, holding up all your shared dreams and plans.

As you both heal from past wounds, your relationship transforms. It's no longer just a mix of two separate histories but a united story full of resilience, understanding, and a robust connection. Sure, it's hard work, but this shared healing journey brings depth and richness to your remarriage that's truly special. It shows you're both ready to face the past with bravery and compassion and build a future full of health, happiness, and love for supporting each other.

The Role of Therapy in Moving Forward

When you're dealing with the rough stuff from past relationships and looking forward to remarrying, therapy can be a real game-changer. Think of it as a guiding light that helps you cut through all the emotional clutter and start fresh. It's not just about taking shelter; it's about setting the stage for a new beginning with some expert help.

Tons of therapy styles act like different routes on a map, guiding you through the terrain of your emotions and thoughts. For example, cognitive behavioral therapy (CBT) helps you spot and change negative thought patterns that mess with your relationships. It's like shining a light on how you think that might be tripping you up, giving you tools to break those destructive cycles and start thinking in ways that support a healthier view of yourself and your relationships.

If you struggle with trust and intimacy because of your past, emotionally focused therapy (EFT) might be your go-to. Based on attachment theory, EFT works through those deep-seated fears of abandonment and insecurity, turning them into ways to connect rather than divide. It's all about understanding your emotional patterns, building empathy and support with your partner, and setting up a remarriage filled with understanding and mutual care.

Narrative therapy is another excellent approach. It lets you and your partner rewrite your life stories, changing narratives colored by past hurts. Think of it as redrawing your map, where you're not victims of your past but heroes of your own story, ready to take on challenges together and build a future of hope and growth.

Therapy isn't just about talking—it's crucial for communication in any relationship. Techniques from the Gottman Method of Couples Therapy, for instance, equip couples with a toolbox for better understanding, respect, and affection. This method builds on the Sound Relationship House Theory, teaching you how to strengthen your relationship by fostering friendship, managing conflict, and creating shared meaning. By improving how you listen, express needs, and handle disagreements, you reinforce your connection and prepare to face life's ups and downs together.

Breaking free from old harmful patterns is a big win in therapy. It's about replacing negative behaviors and thoughts with positive interactions and support. Even though it's tough, the journey through therapy prepares you for a healthier, more loving remarriage. It arms you with insights and tools that help you blend your lives again, ensuring your new chapter is built on solid ground.

Therapy offers guidance, support, and practical tools as you enter a new marriage. It clears up issues that block your heart from loving fully and being loved, making a future filled with understanding, trust, and mutual affection seem achievable. Therapy is your beacon of hope, guiding you and your partner toward a remarriage about emotional health and honest communication.

Transforming Baggage Into Lessons

Turning past heartaches into wisdom is like turning lemons into lemonade—it's all about resilience and making the best out of tricky situations. Instead of just forgetting about past hurts, it's about digging deep and finding the lessons hidden in there. That's where the experiences from past relationships come in handy—they can help you heal and build a stronger foundation for remarriage.

It all starts with looking at things from a different angle. Instead of regretting what went wrong in the past, try seeing it as a learning opportunity. Look hard at your romantic history and be honest about what happened. It might be uncomfortable, but being honest about your role in past relationships can help you see patterns and avoid making the same mistakes in the future.

Once you've identified the areas where you could improve, it's time to turn them into growth opportunities. You may realize that communication was a big issue in your last relationship. Instead of beating yourself up about it, use that insight to work on expressing yourself better. You could read up on effective communication, take workshops on emotional intelligence, or even talk it out in therapy. Addressing these challenges helps you grow personally and sets the stage for a healthier relationship next time.

Applying these lessons in a remarriage is like navigating a river with a better understanding of its currents. By learning from your past mistakes, you can build trust, deepen intimacy, and open those lines of communication. Think of it as proactively taking what you've learned to strengthen your relationship. You could start new rituals to promote honesty and connection or make it a point to check in regularly about how things are going. Whatever it is, you're taking that baggage from the past into a toolkit for building a remarriage about growth and resilience.

But this transformation isn't a one-and-done thing—it's an ongoing process of learning and adapting. Relationships are constantly changing, so it's essential to stay open to feedback from your partner and be willing to adjust your behavior as you grow together. It's all about creating a dynamic marriage that evolves with you and meets your needs.

Sharing this journey with your partner deepens your bond and strengthens your commitment to each other's growth and healing. Together, you're not just merging your lives—creating a future full of promise and potential built on the lessons learned from the past. It's a sacred journey that honors the complexity of the human heart and the enduring power of love to heal, renew, and transform.

Embracing New Beginnings: Celebrating Growth and Transition

We constantly change and evolve, so celebrating our growth is critical. A pause, an acknowledgment of transformation, isn't just a nod to the past. It's a profound statement about what's to come. The soul discovers its rhythm between what's to come and what's to be, aligning what's to be with what's to be.

Certain milestones in growth and healing require a deliberate pause when acknowledging progress and healing. Early in the morning, the sun shines a spotlight on the distance from the shadows. Alternatively, it can take the form of a quiet morning reflection. Intimate shared spaces may also be used to express it, where partners share their journeys and their voices come together to make a whole. Growth milestones aren't celebrated with grand fanfare but rather with profound acknowledgment.

The soul discovers its rhythm between what's to come and what's to be, aligning what's to come with what's to be. We're constantly changing and evolving, so we need to celebrate our growth. A pause, an acknowledgment of change, isn't just a nod to the past. It's a profound statement about what's to come.

Certain milestones must be paused deliberately to acknowledge progress and healing. The shadows of the early morning sun shine brightly. Intimate shared spaces may also be used to express it, where partners share their journeys and their voices come together to make a whole. Growth milestones aren't celebrated with grand fanfare but with profound remembrance.

This evolution manifests itself in rituals of transition, those meticulously crafted ceremonies that tell you what was and what's to come. The soul's readiness to embrace life and love is expressed in these rituals, which are as diverse as the practitioners. Some might escape past entanglements by going on a solitary walk. In anticipation of new beginnings, you might write letters with trembling hands as you say goodbye to old identities and relationships. The old narratives are released by burning them or sealing them up and releasing them into the water. Their ashes fertilize the soil.

Remarriage gives these rituals a collective dimension. This makes them a dance of souls, bringing their narratives into a shared collage of memories for years. It could manifest in creating a vision board with images and words representing the couple's hopes, dreams, and values. It might also be found when planting a garden. This is where each seed sown symbolizes the growth both partners aspire to achieve in themselves and each other. They're not just a merging of paths but a deliberate co-creation of a future vibrant with the colors of mutual growth and understanding.

In this liminal space, where the end of one chapter heralds the optimistic beginning of another, celebrating growth transcends the individual. It becomes a shared narrative of resilience, hope, and boundless possibility. Every tale of loss symbolizes love's capacity to withstand hardship. In addition to recognizing the journey so far, this celebration affirms the future journey. This act adds richness to the story of life, whether it's joy or sorrow. When embraced, this narrative, with all its intricacy and nuances, becomes the most authentic expression of readiness for remarriage. As the story unfolds, there's no need for grand conclusions or summaries because its power lies in the promise of what's yet to be written, the love that grows with each sunrise shared, and the strength forged by starting again.

Preparing Your Heart for a New Love

Getting ready to love someone new is more than just planning a wedding. It's about tuning your heart, mind, and soul to be ready for something real. You want to build a strong foundation for this new chapter.

Being emotionally ready means keeping your heart open. This isn't just about being ready to fall in love or be loved; it's also about facing the vulnerabilities of opening up to someone new. You need a good mix of hope and caution—no need for walls, but maybe some smart boundaries guided by what you've learned from the past. Look at this new relationship with fresh eyes, welcoming what makes it unique without dragging in old disappointments.

A big part of this readiness is loving yourself. Appreciating who you are sets the stage for a successful remarriage. When you value yourself, you bring wholeness into a relationship, not looking for someone else to complete you. This way, both partners can contribute to a relationship about more than the sum of its parts.

Being spiritually ready is also key. It's not necessarily about religion but aligning your core values and beliefs. This step helps you find your ethical or moral direction, guiding you in fostering love, respect, and growth in your new relationship.

And don't forget about keeping hope alive. A positive outlook is essential because it sees the beauty and potential of remarriage. It's about letting go of bitterness from past relationships and staying open to new possibilities for love and shared happiness.

In short, getting ready for a new love is about more than just emotional readiness; it involves cultivating your whole self—your emotions, self-respect, spiritual grounding, and optimism. It's about preparing to marry and engage in a meaningful relationship. This readiness isn't passive; it's about actively preparing yourself for love to take root and flourish.

This whole process—prepping your heart for a new love—is deeply personal yet something many can relate to. It's about setting yourself up for growth, healing, and connection. By focusing on openness, self-love, spiritual alignment, and hope, you're not just stepping into a new marriage but walking into a relationship rich with deep understanding and mutual love.

THREE

Achieving Harmony With Blended Family Dynamics

Blending families involves bringing together people from different backgrounds with past experiences. The challenge is to get everyone working together smoothly. This requires a lot of patience and a deep understanding of each family member's needs and expectations. The goal is to create a setting where everyone can get along and support one another.

Understanding the Complex Dynamics of Blended Families

The key to blending families is understanding that it's a complex situation. Everyone comes with their history and memories. In this new family setup, parents and kids must learn to live together while respecting each other's pasts and working towards a shared future.

Diverse Needs

Imagine a weekend where one child has a soccer game at the same time as another's art exhibition. Managing the logistics and emotional support for each child's interests is challenging. This scenario highlights the importance of making sure everyone in the family feels valued and heard. Recognizing and meeting each family member's unique needs and expectations is crucial.

Communication Strategies

The key is all about working together. Holding a family meeting can be a democratic space where everyone can have a say. Instead of just laying down the rules, these meetings allow for a discussion that respects everyone's viewpoints. Talking over things like household chores and holiday plans, instead of just assigning them, helps build a sense of belonging and mutual respect. This way, everyone can shape the family's story, making the whole process more transparent and empowering.

Adjustment Period

Allowing time for adjustment is crucial. A newly blended family needs nurturing, patience, and time. This adjustment period, full of growing pains, is normal and necessary. It's a time when misunderstandings are more likely. Bonds are tested and gradually strengthened. Recognizing this as a natural phase in blending families helps ease the pressure for instant harmony and sets realistic expectations for building progressively stronger relationships.

Textual Element: Reflection Section

- **Reflect on a Recent Family Meeting.** What topics were easy to discuss, and which were more challenging? Why?
- **Identify Each Family Member's Unique Need or Expectation.** How can these be acknowledged and incorporated into daily family life?

- **Consider a Recent Misunderstanding or Conflict.**
  What root causes can you identify, and how might improved communication strategies address these issues in the future?

The reflection section is about thinking through your blended family's dynamics. Responding to these prompts will help create a nurturing environment where everyone feels valued and heard. It's essential to understand the complex dynamics when blending families. To find harmony, we need to acknowledge everyone's unique background, keep communication open and respectful, and be patient with each other. This approach helps turn a blended family from just a group of people sharing a space into a cohesive unit, celebrating everyone's diversity and growing stronger together.

Stepparenting: Navigating Your Role With Love and Boundaries

Balancing strong support and setting clear boundaries as a stepparent can feel like walking a tightrope. You have to figure out how to build relationships with your stepchildren while respecting the natural boundaries that come with the role. It's about mixing love and discipline to ensure everyone feels respected.

Considering family dynamics and how to support your partner and stepchildren is an excellent way to figure out your role as a stepparent. You must balance being authoritative yet empathetic, offering guidance without overstepping, and giving love that recognizes the complex emotions involved. It's not about imposing yourself but respectfully fitting yourself into the family.

Engaging in activities your stepchildren are passionate about can help build meaningful relationships. Whether it's bonding over music, stargazing, or cooking together, these shared activities can help bridge the gap. These experiences build trust and affection, creating lasting memories.

Regarding discipline, it's essential to be thoughtful and respectful. You should work with your partner to set nurturing limits that align with the family's values rather than imposing your own. This approach reinforces your role as a supportive figure and keeps the biological parent's authority intact. The aim is to create an environment where rules are followed because they are understood and respected, rooted in mutual respect and a shared understanding that they come from a place of love.

Patience, understanding, and love are essential in stepparenting. Navigating this role with care and respect can enrich the family's dynamic.

Creating a United Front: Co-parenting With Ex-Partners

Co-parenting with ex-partners significantly impacts kids' well-being and family harmony. When done right, it can lead to a stable and respectful environment, but it's often filled with challenges. This situation requires building a relationship with your ex focused on raising and caring for your children, not on your past romantic history.

Kids may feel confused and insecure during this time and test the limits. It's crucial to have consistent rules and discipline across both households. Agreeing on a common set of expectations for behavior, routines, and consequences helps keep the child's welfare central to any discussions. It's like agreeing on the rules of a game where everyone knows what to expect, emphasizing the child's overall well-being.

You must communicate clearly and respectfully with your ex to make this work. You should listen actively to understand and empathize, not just argue. Keep these interactions professional, focusing on the kids rather than personal issues. Written agreements about co-parenting plans, regular meetings to adjust these plans, and using mediation services when communication gets tough can all help improve this process.

Presenting a united front is critical to effective co-parenting. It shows the child that they are still surrounded by love and support despite changes. Handle disagreements privately, away from the kids, to give them a consistent, unified message about what you expect and how you support them, which helps maintain security even though their parents live apart.

The main goal of co-parenting with ex-partners is to create a stable environment that supports the child's development, which requires patience, flexibility, and commitment to meet the child's needs first. With consistent rules, clear communication, and a unified approach, co-parenting can successfully address the challenges of blended families. They help kids learn about resolving conflicts and empathy and teach them about maturity and responsibility.

The Kids' Perspective: Supporting Children Through Transition

Blending a family is tough and can be especially hard on the kids. They're trying to navigate a new family dynamic, and listening to their feelings and words is crucial. You must be there with them through this, respecting their pace and views, not just pushing them into a new chapter.

Active listening is essential here. It's more than just hearing words; it's about truly understanding their feelings and showing them that their emotions and concerns are valid by getting down to their level, making eye contact, and creating a space where they feel safe to express themselves. Sometimes, even casual comments from them might hint at deeper worries or needs. By listening actively, you can connect their inner feelings with what's happening in your family's day-to-day life.

Involving them in decisions about everyday things, like picking a movie or decorating a room, makes a big difference, too. It helps them feel part of the family and respect, giving them a say in what happens at home. This isn't just about making them feel included; it's about showing them they're an important part of the family.

Kids in blended families often need support beyond what's at home. Getting them involved in counseling, support groups, or clubs can offer them a broader perspective. Help from others in similar situations can be empowering, giving them a sense of community and tools to handle their feelings and challenges.

In a family where everyone is adjusting, the child's point of view is essential. Listening to their concerns, letting them help make decisions, and connecting them with support systems outside the home can make them feel safe and valued. This approach requires handling the past with much love and creating a family environment where everyone feels united yet free to be themselves. Each kid's unique perspective can strengthen the family as a whole.

Building Bonds: Fostering Connections

Blending families is about building genuine connections based on mutual respect, understanding, and affection. It isn't just about getting along; it's about actively creating a family life that feels right for everyone involved. It takes effort, creativity, patience, and a real commitment to strengthening the ties that hold a family together.

Family activities play a huge part in this process. They provide a setting where everyone can come together to build shared experiences. These could be anything from outdoor adventures that bring out the family's adventurous side to cozy evenings at home filled with stories and laughter. These critical moments turn everyday life into lasting memories and strengthen the bonds between family members.

It's also super important to nurture individual relationships within the family. Each person's history and personality add something special to the family's mix. Family members can connect more deeply by spending one-on-one time with each other. For example, a stepparent might share a love of stargazing with a stepchild, creating memorable moments together looking up at the night sky. Siblings from different parents might discover a shared passion for music, and their impromptu jam sessions may become a new family tradition. These personal connections help everyone feel genuinely part of the family.

Celebrating each family member's achievements and milestones also strengthens the family dynamic. Whether it's a big dinner party for a child's graduation or a quiet congratulation for a stepchild's small win, these celebrations make everyone feel valued. They're not just about acknowledging success but showing that everyone's achievements are essential to the whole family.

Blending families can become a positive, fulfilling experience through love, patience, and mutual respect. While there are challenges in merging lives and traditions, focusing on building both collective and individual relationships can create a family environment that's supportive and resilient. Whether through shared activities, personal bonding time, or celebrating each other's successes, every effort strengthens the family's foundation, making the shared journey one of growth, love, and connection.

Managing Expectations: Reality vs. Fantasy

Blending a family brings excitement and nerves, making it hard to sort out expectations from reality. Finding a balance between optimism and practicality is crucial as you navigate the complex world of blended families, where ideas of instant harmony meet the reality of slow, steady bonding. Patience and understanding are essential for forging deep, meaningful connections.

It's essential to tackle myths about seamlessly merging lives and loves. The myth of instant love paints a picture of immediate bliss but skips over the complex relationship-building needed to blend families. While it's a nice thought that love happens immediately, love grows through shared experiences, nurtured by patience and deepened by understanding. Recognizing this helps set the stage for forming new family bonds that appreciate the various ways people come together.

Patience is a crucial ally in blended families. Just as gardeners understand that flowers take time to bloom, families should embrace the slow and sometimes challenging process of building relationships. Based on realistic expectations, this approach acknowledges that deep connections can't be rushed—they need time and care to develop. Allowing each family member to adjust at their own pace creates a welcoming atmosphere of acceptance and compassion, handling family life's natural ups and downs with ease rather than frustration.

Accepting differences is crucial in managing expectations. Blended families are diverse, and these differences can sometimes cause tension. However, embracing each person's unique traits can enrich the family. Shifting our view to celebrate these differences instead of seeing them as hurdles fosters a culture of inclusion and respect. This acceptance not only defines the family's identity but also highlights the beauty of diversity and the power of love to connect us.

Living in a blended family involves balancing reality with expectations and debunking myths with the truths of many families' experiences. Embracing patience, nurturing relationships over time, and celebrating each family member's uniqueness is critical. Love and connection in a blended family unfold gradually, woven together by shared experiences, mutual respect, and unwavering support—it's about building a strong, loving family, not achieving perfection.

Holidays and Traditions: Creating New Memories Together

Blended family life mixes old and new holidays and traditions, creating a unique blend of memories that link the past with the present. These occasions are not just fun; they also balance respecting old customs while introducing new ones. This mix helps families craft their identity by combining personal backgrounds with shared experiences into something everyone can call their own.

Getting everyone involved in planning and celebrating holidays isn't just about being fair; it's about making each person feel valued. It turns planning into a fun activity full of anticipation and excitement. Picture a family cooking a holiday meal where every dish represents a different family tradition or decorating the living room with items that reflect various cultural heritages. These efforts make everyone's voice matter and build a sense of belonging.

Honoring important traditions from each family member's past is crucial. It's about carefully blending these memories into the new family culture without losing sight of their origins. Maybe it's about merging two holiday meals into one big celebration that honors both or mixing up the music playlists to keep things fresh yet familiar. This way, families respect their roots while celebrating their new life together.

Forming lasting positive memories is critical to shaping a family's identity. These aren't just random moments; they're the ones that stick, like impromptu dance parties on a weeknight, marathon board game sessions that end in laughter, or quiet afternoons making crafts together. These memories deepen family bonds and give everyone a sense of unity and belonging.

By creating meaningful traditions and new experiences, blended families build a rich tapestry of life full of joy, warmth, and lasting connections. Planning with everyone in mind, honoring each person's heritage, and making new memories together show the beauty of unity in diversity and the strength of shared experiences, all wrapped in love.

Addressing Resistance and Rejection in Blended Families

When family members face the challenges of adjusting to a new family setup, it's common for resistance and rejection to show up. These reactions are often rooted in deep worries and insecurities about the changes. It's essential to see these feelings not as roadblocks but as opportunities to deepen understanding and strengthen relationships within the family.

You must examine the psychological reasons behind these behaviors to understand why someone might resist or reject family changes. For example, a new marriage might make kids worry about losing their spot in a parent's heart or feel like accepting a stepparent is betraying their other parent. What looks like resistance or rejection is often just a way for them to protect themselves from these fears.

It's important to be sensitive and patient when helping struggling family members. Open conversations can make a difference. Creating a safe space to discuss their fears, concerns, and hopes regarding the new family setup can help address more profound issues. These discussions should focus on validating feelings and thoughtfully addressing concerns.

Finding common interests or activities can help everyone connect in a relaxed way, breaking down barriers. It's also good to involve everyone in creating new family traditions, showing that the new family is about adding to their lives, not taking anything away.

Sometimes, deeper issues might be at play if the resistance or rejection keeps up. Professional help, like family therapy, can be valuable. Therapy can guide families through the challenges of blending lives, providing tools and strategies tailored to their situation. This support can pave the way for better communication, understanding, and empathy among family members.

Dealing with resistance and rejection builds trust, empathy, and respect. Behind every act of resistance or rejection, there's often a call for reassurance or a desire to feel included and understood. If blended families approach these challenges with open hearts and minds, they can transform potential conflicts into chances to grow closer. By taking the time to understand each family member's feelings and fostering connections, the family can create a supportive environment where everyone feels valued and accepted.

The Importance of One-on-One Time With Each Child

Blended families are complex networks where every connection counts. Dedicating time to each child is vital because it strengthens their bond with the family and shows them they matter.

Each child is different, influenced by their experiences and dreams, so you must tailor how you engage with them. For instance, one child might need lots of reassurance, while another might be looking for more adventurous activities that can be shared safely with a parent.

Spending one-on-one time with them lets us meet their specific needs, making them feel valued and secure.

The foundation of these individual relationships is trust, which isn't just given; it's built through consistently showing up and being reliable. Quiet moments spent together to build mutual respect and understanding. This trust is crucial and comes from every conversation, secret shared, and dream supported.

The activities for these one-on-one times vary, making each interaction unique. It could be a morning jog where you talk about everything from small daily stuff to more significant, deeper topics or doing a project together, like building a model airplane or fixing something around the house. These moments allow the child to be themselves and explore new parts of who they are while feeling their parent's full support and attention.

This focused time is more than just hanging out; it's a way to celebrate the child's individuality and directly respond to their needs. It's about building trust and fostering deep connections that are vital for integrating the family as a whole.

These individual times help each child feel important and enrich the family dynamic, adding layers of understanding, empathy, and respect. They make every family member feel like a vital part of the group, which is crucial for creating a harmonious blended family. It's not just a nice extra; it's essential for nurturing deep, trusting relationships and a sense of belonging.

Spending one-on-one time with each child in a blended family is about much more than doing activities together; it's about building a network of connection and understanding that celebrates each person's uniqueness while bringing everyone closer together.

The Long-Term Journey of Blending Families

Blended families need more time to work through their complexities than we often see in quick media snapshots or short stories. It's about building shared experiences and understanding over time, not just in brief moments. Appreciating how long it takes for deep connections to form and for different lives to mesh together helps make this journey a source of strength.

A crucial part of surviving this lengthy process is adopting a growth mindset. This mindset views challenges not as obstacles that can't be overcome but as opportunities to strengthen family ties. This mindset encourages flexibility and resilience, helping everyone see challenges as chances to grow closer rather than reasons to give up. Whether facing tough times or adapting to new situations, there's a lot of personal and collective growth if everyone is open to dealing with these complexities.

Celebrating both small and significant achievements is crucial. Every step forward, whether managing to enjoy the holidays together or resolving a complex conflict, demonstrates how the family is growing closer and becoming more assertive. These moments of celebration, big or small, highlight the progress everyone is making by putting in the time and effort. It's important to remember that blending a family isn't about making huge changes overnight but gradually building trust and strengthening ties.

All this takes a lot of effort and shows how dynamic a blended family's life can be. It requires patience and understanding—necessary traits, not just nice to have. Building these relationships takes time, and everyone involved needs to commit to the long haul. Continuously nurturing understanding and empathy within the family helps ensure the family can handle the ups and downs of coming together.

As you tell the story of your blended family, you'll see how the mix of different experiences and viewpoints makes everything richer. Over time, this blend creates a complex but beautiful harmony woven through shared experiences and a commitment to supporting each other. This ongoing story isn't just about overcoming challenges; it's about growing together and finding joy in being a family.

This journey with a blended family is full of ongoing lessons—about sticking together, learning from challenges, and celebrating together. These lessons guide us toward a loving, growing, and harmonious family life.

FOUR

Navigating Relationships With Ex-Partners

Relationships with ex-partners can change over time, bringing challenges and growth chances. It's really important to set and keep healthy boundaries in these relationships. These boundaries help keep things stable and ensure everyone knows what to expect. Clear and respectful boundaries support an environment where kids can do well, and new marriages can strengthen.

Establishing Healthy Boundaries With Ex-Partners

Setting boundaries with ex-partners is challenging but necessary. These boundaries help ensure the kids are okay and your new relationship stays stable. They also act as clear rules about how everyone should interact and their responsibilities, helping keep things smooth and predictable.

Boundary Examples

Think about how you handle communication. To keep things clear and have a record, decide that all messages about the kids should go through a specific channel, like email or a co-parenting app. A shared calendar between homes can help the kids know what to expect and feel more settled about visits. Also, when it comes to big decisions about things like education or health, it's helpful to have clear agreements about who gets involved and how you'll make those final decisions. This can help cut down on conflicts.

Enforcing Boundaries

Enforcing these boundaries requires a mix of firmness and flexibility. It's all about clearly communicating the boundaries and being open to adjusting them as needed. The goal is to find a balance where the boundaries are respected without being so strict that they cause unnecessary conflict.

Navigating Challenges

When boundaries are tested, it's important to respond thoughtfully instead of reacting on impulse. For example, if an ex-partner skips the usual communication channels, which is confusing, it's a good idea to review that boundary. You can discuss why this breach happened and devise a solution that respects everyone's needs, especially the kids'.

Textual Element: Reflection Section

- **Reflect on your current boundaries with ex-partners.** Are they clear, respected, and influential?
- **Consider a recent instance where a boundary was tested.** How was it handled, and what could be improved?
- **Think about the channels of communication open between you and your ex-partner.** Are they conducive to constructive exchanges, or is there room for improvement?

Setting and maintaining boundaries is key to managing relationships with ex-partners effectively. It requires patience, understanding, and adapting to keep the family environment stable and peaceful.

Effective Communication Strategies for Co-parenting

Setting and maintaining clear boundaries can make a big difference in keeping things smooth when dealing with ex-partners. It's about ensuring everyone's on the same page, which leads to a happier, more harmonious family life. Being patient, understanding, adaptable, and skilled at using the right tools and strategies are key.

For managing the day-to-day, many digital tools and platforms are designed explicitly for co-parenting. These can help streamline everything from scheduling to communication about the kids. Consider how useful an app designed for co-parenting could be: messages sorted by topic, updates shared instantly, and expenses tracked transparently. This setup helps keep things clear and focused on what's important—raising kids together but apart.

It's crucial to keep the kids' well-being at the forefront. Every decision or message considers how it affects the children. It's about cutting through the clutter and focusing on supporting them, like sharing updates about school activities, personal achievements, or funny little moments. This approach helps maintain a sense of partnership in parenting, even when you're no longer together.

Conflict is inevitable, but how you handle it makes all the difference. When disagreements pop up, it's better to take a moment to think before responding. Thinking helps prevent the situation from escalating. Listening to understand each other rather than arguing can foster empathy and make it easier to work through issues. The goal isn't to "win" but to find the best solutions for the kids.

In essence, effectively managing co-parenting communication involves using the right tools, prioritizing your kids' needs, and handling conflicts with a cool head. Ex-partners can effectively support their kids by focusing on these areas, ensuring a stable and supportive co-parenting relationship.

Navigating Financial Responsibilities With Ex-Partners

Handling money matters in co-parenting setups hinges on transparency about who's responsible for what. This clarity is key for keeping things smooth after a divorce. You establish legal agreements outlining who pays for child support, school costs, and health expenses. It's not just paperwork; it's a roadmap that keeps everyone on the same page and makes things predictable and fair for the kids.

But life changes, and so might the parents' financial situations. When that happens, it's important to discuss and update the agreements, such as adjusting how much one pays in child support or rethinking contributions to college funds. It's all about staying flexible and keeping the lines of communication open to ensure the financial plan keeps working for everyone involved, especially the kids.

Being open about these financial duties with any new partner is also crucial. These aren't just leftovers from a previous relationship but ongoing commitments to your kids. Being upfront about this can strengthen a new relationship. You might need to explain how these obligations fit into your current financial planning and how you and your new partner can handle them together. Keeping this dialogue honest and ongoing means these responsibilities won't sneak up on you but will be part of the shared life you're building.

Managing money with an ex involves clear agreements, flexibility, and transparency. It's complex, sure, but by focusing on these elements, you can ensure the kids are well cared for, keep respect high between co-parents, and lay a strong foundation for new relationships. Seeing these financial responsibilities as a part of your role as a parent, not just a burden, helps transform co-parenting into a tangible demonstration of commitment and care.

The Impact of New Relationships on Co-Parenting Dynamics

Co-parenting becomes more complex when new relationships enter the picture. These changes mean everyone involved has to adjust and think over their roles, responsibilities, and boundaries to keep things stable for the kids while adapting to new family dynamics. Handling this well means being careful about human emotions and working towards a setup that works for everyone.

Introducing new partners to your kids and ex should be done carefully, ensuring it's the right time and you're considering the kids' feelings. Introduce new partners gradually in relaxed settings to avoid making anyone feel uncomfortable or pressured. This slow approach helps build trust and connection.

Respecting boundaries is crucial, especially about how new partners fit into co-parenting roles. This means that biological parents should keep making the big decisions about their kids' lives. The new partner's role should grow based on everyone's comfort levels, especially the kids', ensuring they feel secure and that their primary relationships are still solid.

Adjusting your expectations as things change is vital. Being flexible and open to discussing how things are evolving can help you refigure co-parenting setups as relationships with new partners develop. This doesn't weaken co-parenting; it enriches it by ensuring it fits the family's current situation while respecting past relationships and looking forward to what's next.

Navigating new relationships while co-parenting comes down to being patient, understanding, and always thinking about what's best for the kids. It's about balancing between setting clear boundaries and being flexible with how family dynamics change. Always communicate honestly and empathetically. When you manage this balance well, co-parenting can become a dynamic and supportive network that helps the whole family grow closer and stronger.

Protecting Your Remarriage From External Stresses

Remarriage is complex, especially when former partners and new relationships mix. It's all about being resilient, loving deeply, and committing fully. You must also be smart about keeping the relationship strong against external pressures, especially when dealing with co-parenting and interactions with ex-partners. Showing a united front is crucial, as is communicating openly and ensuring you care for yourself to keep your marriage solid.

United Front

Showing a united front lays down the law about unity and resilience. Sticking together through thick and thin is crucial when rebuilding a family. You've got to be on the same page when making decisions about the kids, maintaining consistent rules and boundaries, and handling issues with ex-partners together. You must ensure your actions and decisions reflect your shared goals and values. Even when you disagree, presenting a united front is important, especially to your kids and former partners. A united front helps protect your marriage from external stresses and creates a stable and peaceful home environment that gives your kids a sense of security.

Communication

Effective communication is critical to clearing up misunderstandings and confusion in relationships. Remarriage strengthens the bond between partners, helping them connect more emotionally. It's essential to be brave about voicing concerns, open about sharing fears, and willing to discuss co-parenting challenges without feeling threatened. The goal is to create a safe space where conversations aren't about conflict but about bridging gaps and overcoming external pressures together. This way, any challenges with ex-partners become something you handle together, using your partnership's collective wisdom and strength.

Self-Care and Support

Handling co-parenting demands and issues with ex-partners can be challenging when blending families, but taking care of yourself and leaning on support can make a big difference. Staying healthy in a remarriage depends on how well each person takes care of themselves. Self-care is more than just treating yourself; it's about keeping your mind, body, and spirit in good shape to stay strong against outside stress. You might enjoy a quiet walk in the morning, writing to clear your head, or doing something you love that rejuvenates you. These activities help keep you centered so you can approach co-parenting and interactions with ex-partners calmly and clearly.

But it's not just about self-care. Having a solid support system is crucial, too—getting empathy from counseling, solidarity from support groups, or understanding from family and friends. These connections provide comfort from shared experiences and insights from collective wisdom, which can make the remarriage journey smoother and more fulfilling.

Protecting your relationship from external pressures is essential by presenting a united front, keeping communication open, and committing to self-care and strong support networks. These strategies help build a resilient family unit ready to face life's challenges together. By focusing on these critical areas, your remarriage can rise above the complications and be a strong, united, and proactive partnership.

Handling Conflict with Ex-Partners Gracefully

Conflicts are common when dealing with an ex-partner, especially when kids are involved. Think of handling these conflicts as trying to keep things calm and constructive. This approach helps you work through disagreements smoothly and keeps co-parenting cooperative.

When a conflict arises, the first step is to calm things down. This requires quick thinking, patience, and smart-talking. If you can cool off before responding, it helps you think clearly. Understanding where the other person comes from can make a potentially challenging situation more manageable. Acknowledging the other person's concerns, like saying, "I see this is important to you," can move the conversation from a fight to teamwork.

Keeping the kids' best interests in mind when dealing with these disagreements is crucial rather than trying to win the argument. Decide what's essential for the kids and what's not. Not every disagreement needs to be a battle; sometimes, it's okay to let things go, find a middle ground, or revisit the issue later.

If you're stuck and can't sort things out between yourselves, bringing in a mediator or attorney might be a good move. They're good at staying neutral and can help you find solutions that might not be obvious because of all the emotions involved. Getting this kind of help doesn't mean you've failed; it just shows you when it's time to get extra support to keep things fair and focused on what's best for the kids.

Managing co-parenting conflicts well is essential. You can handle these situations with maturity by staying calm, choosing your battles wisely, and sometimes getting outside help. This way, you keep the peace and build a supportive and stable environment for your kids, showing them that even though things can get tricky, you can handle it with grace and cooperation.

Legal Considerations in Co-Parenting Arrangements

As co-parents, we juggle different responsibilities and rights, which can get confusing, especially with kids involved. Knowing the ins and outs helps. It gives you the clarity and foresight to handle the complexities of co-parenting effectively.

Understanding Rights and Responsibilities

Having a clear plan that spells out each parent's rights and responsibilities is critical to handling the legal side of co-parenting. This plan ensures the kids' welfare is always the focus, detailing who gets the kids when, who decides on big issues like education and healthcare, and how the financial responsibilities are split. For example, a legal custody agreement will lay out which parent makes important decisions about the child's life, and physical custody arrangements specify where the kids live and how much time they spend with each parent. Knowing these legal details helps parents manage co-parenting with more confidence.

Modifying Agreements

As your family evolves, so should your legal agreements—especially if big changes like moving, shifts in financial status, or new family members joining the fold. When these changes occur, assessing the situation carefully and adjusting your legal documents is crucial. To update your agreements, you must show that these changes significantly affect your child's well-being. Often, this process is guided by a lawyer to make sure everything is done right. This step is a reminder of how family life can change and how legal arrangements need to be flexible to keep up with these changes, whether that means going to court or just updating your records.

Protecting the New Family Unit

Protecting your new family setup becomes a top priority when you remarry, including handling legal stuff smartly while respecting your co-parenting duties. You need to get a good grip on legal tools like prenuptial agreements, which help spell out financial responsibilities and safeguard assets for all kids involved, including biological and stepchildren. Considerating these kids' preferences in your estate planning is crucial. These steps are more than just paperwork; they're essential supports that help keep your blended family's intentions clear and their legal rights protected.

Handling co-parenting arrangements requires staying sharp, planning, and always putting the kids first. It's a path where knowing the ins and outs of the law helps keep things smooth, adjustments are made as life changes, and safeguards keep the family's structure solid. The aim is to maintain harmony, stability, and growth through well-understood rules. Essentially, building a family life on a foundation of mutual understanding, respect, and care, despite its complexities and inevitable changes, is what it's all about.

Supporting Your Partner in Co-Parenting Challenges

When two people come together with their backgrounds and hopes for the future, it shows how resilient and flexible we can be. Throw co-parenting into the mix, and things get even trickier because now you're navigating relationships beyond just the two of you. Supporting your partner means understanding each other emotionally. Your blended family needs a strong foundation of support from both of you. This means handling things carefully and sticking together no matter what.

Listening and Empathy

When you support your partner, it's not just about hearing them out —it's about understanding where they're coming from with an open heart and a ready spirit. Good support digs deep, getting to the core of what they feel and experience. By listening this way, you get a glimpse of the world through their eyes, which helps you offer meaningful support that respects their complex journey. Their experiences, especially those involving ex-partners or decisions about the kids, add layers to their story that you must consider as you both navigate this path together.

Navigating Your Role

Co-parenting is like walking a path already shaped by those who've walked it. Supporting your partner here means understanding your role in this complex picture. Knowing the boundaries is crucial to ensure your actions and words uplift and don't overstep. Your job is to support your partner without getting in the way of their primary co-parenting responsibilities, which are crucial for the kids' well-being.

Finding a way to add positively to the co-parenting situation means offering insights that help more than they confuse and being there in a way that comforts without intruding. Achieving this balance comes from open conversations with your partner and a joint commitment to handle this challenge together. This approach ensures your support is helpful and respectful, strengthening your partnership and the family dynamics.

United Approach

Handling co-parenting legalities takes patience, foresight, and a strong focus on what's best for the kids. Legal setups help guide us, but we must stay adaptable as life changes and ensure everyone's protection. Laws help set the ground rules and keep things stable and harmonious. With all their twists and turns, families are fundamentally about understanding and respecting each other, built on caring and shared goals. It's all about keeping open lines of communication, resolving differences, and always putting the kids' happiness and safety first.

As you, your partner, and the whole co-parenting crew roll with life's changes, remember it's an evolving process. A united, flexible approach rooted in respect and understanding doesn't just shield us from stress and allows our family to grow, love, and stay stable.

Even though our actions and challenges are different in this complicated journey, our main goal is always the same: to be stable, caring, and dedicated. By listening to each other, being considerate in our roles, and facing challenges together, we do more than keep our relationship stable while co-parenting; we create a family environment that flourishes despite the obstacles. We discover our strength, purpose, and way forward as a team.

The Role of Mediation in Co-Parenting Conflicts

Co-parenting conflicts can pop up and mess with communication and teamwork. Mediation can help here by offering a neutral place where you can sort out these issues and find solutions that work for everyone. It creates an atmosphere where everyone can understand each other better and work together, which is great for everyone involved, especially the kids.

The Benefits of Mediation

A mediator is trained to handle family conflicts and helps facilitate conversations between co-parents. This way, disagreements become chances for growth and understanding instead of fights. Mediation strengthens family relationships because it's less aggressive than going to court. Mediation allows for solutions that fit a family's needs, unlike the standard solutions that courts often provide. Everyone can discuss their needs and worries in mediation without fearing backlash or judgment. When co-parents collaborate to develop a resolution, they're more likely to follow through.

The Mediation Process Unveiled

When you start mediation, the mediator will first lay down some ground rules to ensure everyone talks openly and respectfully. In these sessions, the mediation process is tailored to fit the needs of the co-parents, making it both structured and adaptable. The mediator then helps facilitate the discussion, ensuring everyone can speak and steering the conversation away from blame. They help highlight the main issues and guide co-parents in thinking through possible solutions, always keeping the kids' perspectives and needs in mind. This team effort in solving problems wraps up with writing down an agreement. This agreement isn't legally binding on its own, but it can form the basis of a court order, which makes it enforceable.

Preparing for Mediation

Preparing for mediation is like preparing for a big event—ensuring every discussion is clear and on point is crucial. It's a good idea to talk through your goals for the mediation for yourself and your family. Knowing what you want and need before you start is key. Gather any important documents you might need, like financial records or past communication logs, to keep things grounded. Approaching mediation with an open mind and a readiness to compromise increases your chances of finding a resolution that works for everyone. This open approach helps build mutual understanding, especially when everyone prioritizes the kids' well-being.

Co-parenting mixes many old and new emotions and challenges. Mediation shows how dialogue, understanding, and compromise can help navigate these complexities. It's important to stay patient and open to finding solutions that work for everyone and will last over time. Mediation is a respectful way to handle conflicts, looking out for everyone's dignity and needs. When you commit to mediation, you're investing in the hope that you can work through your differences in a way that's good for your kids.

Keeping the Focus on the Children's Well-Being

Co-parenting is about the kids—keeping their well-being and interests at the forefront. It's about more than just saying you're putting them first; you've got to commit to looking after their emotional health and needs.

The best way to handle co-parenting decisions is to consider how things will affect the kids. This means considering their emotional and psychological needs along with their physical ones. For example, choose a place to live that keeps their school and social life stable or make sure they feel comfortable expressing their feelings about the co-parenting setup.

Listening to what kids have to say is crucial. It shows them they're valued and that their opinions matter. This helps them open up about their worries and wishes and teaches them that their thoughts are important. Finding the right balance between encouraging them to express themselves and ensuring they're okay can be challenging.

It's also important to show kids how to handle relationships respectfully and civilly, especially in tough situations like divorce or separation. Kids are always watching and learning how to manage emotions and conflicts by seeing how their parents do it. If they see you handling things respectfully, even when you disagree, they'll pick up some great skills for their relationships.

Focusing on the kids helps make sense of co-parenting, especially when old relationship issues come into play. You can build a stable and nurturing co-parenting environment by always putting the kids' needs first, staying open to what they say, and leading by example with respect.

As we wrap up this discussion, remember that co-parenting is fundamentally about what's best for the kids. By focusing on their needs, actively listening to them, and showing them how to handle relationships respectfully, you're setting them up for a future where they can thrive emotionally. This approach isn't just about managing co-parenting; it's about fostering a loving and supportive atmosphere in your blended family, ensuring respect and understanding are at the heart of everything you do.

Comprehensive Guide to Remarriage Success

CREATE A STRONG MARITAL BASE, BLEND FAMILIES, FOSTER ENDURING CONNECTIONS, AND SHAPE A SHARED FUTURE

"True love doesn't happen right away; it's an ever-growing process."

Ricardo Montalban

Hey there! I'm Taylor Reed, your guide on this transformative journey of remarriage. Like you, I once faced the uncertainty and excitement of blending lives and families, which inspired me to dive deep into the dynamics of successful remarriages. I've turned my discoveries into a passion and made it my mission to make remarriage a rewarding experience for everyone, no matter their background. I believe in the power of love to build bridges, and I'm committed to helping you and your partner create a thriving, resilient union.

You might wonder, "Is remarriage that different from the first time?" Let's tackle that question head-on. Remarriage does bring unique challenges, such as blending families and aligning established lives, but it also offers incredible opportunities for growth and happiness. Imagine having a guide that helps you manage these complexities effectively, allowing you and your partner to focus on what you do best—building a life filled with love, understanding, and mutual growth.

Now, I need your help. Reviews are crucial because they help other people decide whether this book is right for them—especially when it comes to something as important as building a successful remarriage. Here's my ask for the countless couples out there you've never met:

Please help them by leaving a review for this book.

It costs nothing and takes less than a minute, but your words could make a difference. Your review could help:

- ...one more couple finds harmony in their blended family.
- ...one more spouse understands and connects with their partner.
- ...one more family navigates their challenges with confidence.
- ...one more couple reinforces their commitment to each other.
- ...one more love story to flourish and grow.

To share your thoughts and make a difference, just scan the QR code below to leave your review:

If you enjoy helping others, you're exactly who I'm looking to connect with. Welcome to the community! I'm excited to help you navigate your remarriage journey and can't wait to share strategies that will strengthen your relationship.

Thank you from the bottom of my heart. Now, let's get back to building those lasting connections.

Your biggest fan,
Taylor Reed

P.S. Sharing valuable advice makes you a key part of someone else's journey. Please pass this book on if you believe it will benefit another couple.

FIVE

Creating Harmony Through Communication

O ur relationships lean a lot on what we say and don't say. Getting good at this communication is super important in a remarriage. This chapter digs into the different layers of how we talk to each other, looking at the little things that shape our chats. We'll cover how to adjust our communication, use emotional intelligence, and effectively give and receive feedback. These skills can turn regular conversations into deep connections when we use them right.

Advanced Communication Skills for Couples

Effective communication is more than just talking; it means understanding how each other communicates. For things to go smoothly, partners must adjust to each other's talking and listening methods.

Tailoring Communication

You can overcome communication barriers by changing your approach to match your partner's style. Adjust how you talk based on how your partner feels, choose the best times to have conversations, and think about how you phrase things. For instance, talking about important family matters during a quiet walk instead of in the hectic morning can make the discussion smoother and more effective.

Emotional Intelligence

Emotional intelligence guides how we communicate with our partner, helping us understand their emotions and nonverbal signals. It's about noticing the small things, like if their eyebrows furrow, their shoulders tense up, or they sigh quietly. Understanding what these signs mean is critical. Emotional intelligence involves seeing these cues and reacting in ways that show you get it. A simple touch, a pause in the conversation, or changing the topic can all show you care and understand.

Feedback Loops

Positive feedback loops in communication are crucial because they help relationships grow. They happen when you show appreciation for your partner's practical communication efforts. For example, saying something like, "I appreciate how you listened to my concerns about moving," after a discussion reinforces good communication habits. This acknowledgment makes your partner feel valued and motivates them to keep up the good work in future conversations.

Textual Element: Reflection Section

- **Reflect on a recent conversation with your partner.**
  Were there moments when adjusting your communication style could have enhanced the exchange?
- **Think about a time when recognizing a nonverbal cue from your partner changed the course of a**

conversation. What did you notice, and how did you respond?

- **Consider the feedback loops in your communication.** How often do you acknowledge and appreciate your partner's effective communication efforts?

Remarriage mixes past experiences with current realities, making top-notch communication skills crucial. Understanding nonverbal cues through emotional intelligence and building positive feedback loops can significantly improve your relationship. These methods help exchange information effectively and enrich connections, deepening bonds and creating a peaceful environment within the complexities of a blended family.

Conflict Resolution: Navigating Disagreements With Love

Disagreements might feel like roadblocks, but if you handle them with love, compassion, and a genuine desire to work things out, they can help your relationship grow and strengthen. In remarriage, where you're blending past experiences with future hopes, being good at resolving conflicts shows how strong your relationship is.

Diverse Landscapes of Conflict

Conflicts vary a lot. Some are small, everyday bumps that you can smooth over with little tweaks here and there. Others are big, at the core of what you and your partner believe or dream about. Then there are all those disagreements, each unique and needing its approach. It's not about dodging conflicts; it's about understanding each one and dealing with it to keep you and your relationship healthy.

The Art of the Cooling-Off Period

When disagreements heat up, it's easy for words to turn into weapons. That's why taking a break is so important—it's a chance to let the storm of initial reactions calm down and give room for more thoughtful responses. It's not about avoiding the issue but about organizing your thoughts, cooling down, and returning to tackle the problem calmly. Taking this break can help clarify the argument and show ways to sort things out that you might not see when emotions run high.

Charting a Course Toward Solutions

Understanding the situation and aiming for the proper outcomes is critical to resolving conflicts when you hit a snag. Shifting the focus to solutions helps move the conversation from pointing fingers to understanding each other. This approach doesn't pit partners against each other but looks for answers considering both sides' needs and desires. By openly discussing the issue and brainstorming together, the solutions you come up with are compromises and real resolutions that strengthen the relationship for the future.

In these moments, it becomes clear that the real issue isn't the person you love but the conflict itself. When you tackle the problem together, you turn a potential divide into a chance for growth, better understanding, and closeness. Every resolved disagreement paves the way for a stronger relationship, tested by challenges but solidified with care and understanding.

When you blend past experiences with new challenges, being good at resolving conflicts shows a deep commitment to sticking together and growing. By facing these challenges together, your relationship becomes a space of mutual respect, affection, and support. Instead of fearing disagreements, you start to see them as chances to deepen your connection, knowing that with each issue you overcome, your bond grows stronger.

The Importance of Vulnerability in Deepening Connections

When you remarry, there are dreams, hopes, and fears that usually don't get talked about. Opening up about these personal thoughts with your partner is about vulnerability. While many see vulnerability as a weakness, it's a strength in a healthy relationship. Sharing these deeper feelings builds trust and strengthens your connection, bringing you closer and helping you understand each other better. But it's important to balance how open you are with keeping healthy emotional boundaries, which can be tricky to navigate.

Sharing Fears and Dreams

Just think about how great it would be if everyone was open and just got each other. Sharing your deepest fears and dreams with someone goes beyond just talking; it's like letting them into the most private parts of who you are. You're showing them everything that excites you and everything that scares you. Doing this takes a unique environment where there's no judgment, just a lot of empathy. In this space, it's not about trying to fix things or throw out advice. It's about being there and hearing what the other person is saying. Sure, it's risky to open up like this, but it's worth it because it brings people closer together, helping bridge the gap between what we experience and how we see things.

Building Trust

Trust is the bedrock of any solid relationship, especially when it's built on being open with each other. A deep trust comes from knowing your partner respects and values your openness. When both of you can be vulnerable together, it feels like you're part of something special—where fears aren't mocked, and dreams aren't brushed off, but instead, they're cherished. This shared openness deepens your trust, not just in each other's compassion but also in the strength of the bond it creates. Even when doubts and conflicts arise, this trust reminds you of the safe space you've built, rooted in understanding and acceptance.

Vulnerability Without Overexposure

Being open with your partner doesn't mean you have to share everything at once. It's about slowly letting your guard down in a way that respects both the depth of your relationship and your boundaries. Start by reflecting on what you're comfortable sharing, then establish clear boundaries. Think of it as gradually getting to know each other deeper, layer by layer, while keeping some things back until you feel comfortable and trust has been established. This approach ensures that becoming vulnerable with each other strengthens your bond without causing emotional overload.

Showing your true self to your partner is powerful. It allows you to build a stronger connection that's also mindful of maintaining healthy emotional limits. By sharing your innermost fears and dreams and carefully managing how you navigate these personal revelations, you can turn your relationship into a place of mutual understanding, support, and profound closeness.

The Key to Understanding Your Partner

Active listening is the key to understanding your partner. It's about tuning in, not just hearing your partner out. When actively listening, you focus entirely, understand what's being said, and respond thoughtfully. This kind of listening goes beyond words; it's about picking up on what isn't said aloud, like those subtle emotions hidden under the surface. Doing this builds a deeper connection and understanding with your partner, making understanding where they're coming from easier.

Techniques for Effective Active Listening

When you get the hang of active listening, you start to pick up on a lot more. Noticing the little things, like how someone might look away when unsure or drop their shoulders when they're tired, helps you get what's being said—even the stuff that's not out loud. You show you get it by nodding, reaching out for a gentle touch, or just mimicking their expressions, which opens the door for even more honesty between you two.

Throwing in a few words like "I see," "I understand," or "Tell me more" does wonders, too. It's not just about making the other person feel heard; it's about creating a connection and showing them they matter. These small nods during a chat can take your conversation to a new level of closeness and trust.

The Crucial Element of Undivided Attention

Giving your partner your full attention shows your commitment and respect, especially in a world of distractions. Active listening means fully focusing on them—turning off your phone, ignoring notifications, and stopping your inner monologue to be entirely in the moment. When you cut out all the external and internal noise, your conversations can go deeper, building a stronger connection and understanding.

The Subtleties of Reflective Listening

Listening to your partner and reflecting on their words helps clarify and validate their thoughts and feelings. This part of active listening involves listening carefully and then paraphrasing their words or describing their emotions. You might start your reflection by saying, "So, what I'm hearing is..." or "It sounds like you're feeling...". This lets your partner see that you're trying to understand them. By mirroring their words, you show that you're fully engaged, and it helps your partner hear their thoughts from another perspective, which can provide clarity and reveal deeper emotions or ideas they hadn't fully articulated yet.

Active listening is essential, where understanding each other is key. It's more than just being quiet while the other person is talking; it involves engaging, paying attention to what they say and don't say, and being ready to show that you get it. This kind of listening involves picking up on nonverbal cues, offering words of affirmation, giving your full attention, and using reflective techniques. When you genuinely listen in this way, you open up deeper levels of understanding and connection, making every conversation an opportunity to strengthen your bond. Active listening becomes a beautiful, transformative part of your relationship, blending experiences, emotions, and hopes into a harmonious life.

Negotiation Skills for a Harmonious Marriage

In remarriage, negotiation is key. It's not just about hashing things out; it's about finding ways to respect and make each other happy. Negotiations aim for win-win solutions where both partners feel their needs and desires are met. This approach turns individual wants into collective wins, requiring empathy and a strong commitment to what's best for both of you. For example, when picking a vacation spot, you aim to find a place that satisfies your thrill-seeking and your partner's need to unwind. It's about making choices that make you happy and build shared experiences.

However, reaching these agreements means making compromises or even sacrifices. It's crucial to know the difference between the two. A healthy compromise means adjusting your wants to find a happy middle ground and strengthening the relationship. But sacrifice is trickier—it happens when one partner's needs overshadow the other's, which can hurt the relationship if it happens too often.

You'll need a whole set of negotiation skills to handle this well. Active listening is like a tool that helps you understand what your partner needs and why. It turns the negotiation into a joint effort to meet a common goal instead of a battle. Another handy tool is using "I" statements, which keep the conversation calm and focused on feelings rather than accusations.

So, negotiating in remarriage isn't about winning a fight; it's an opportunity to deepen your connection and ensure you can chase your dreams together. It's about using your negotiation skills to create an atmosphere of love and mutual respect, where every decision helps you grow closer and build a good life for both of you.

Addressing Sensitive Topics

Navigating sensitive topics like finances, intimacy, and parenting in a relationship can be tricky. These are areas loaded with emotions and potential for misunderstanding. Handling these topics with your partner requires careful consideration, much like dealing with something precious and delicate. It's about building and testing the strength of your relationship.

To start these discussions, create an environment that helps you open up. Choose a quiet place and time where distractions won't interrupt your conversation, and maybe add some soft background music to help set a calm, open mood. This setting should feel like a safe space where you can talk honestly.

The way you talk to each other matters a lot here. Using "I" statements can change the whole tone of the conversation. Instead of saying, "You always do this," say, "I feel this way when this happens." This makes a big difference because it helps keep the conversation about understanding each other rather than blaming.

It's important to let go of preconceived notions regarding tough topics like money, how close you feel, or parenting. It's about looking at what you both want and need from the relationship, not just sticking rigidly to your point of view. Finding common ground can help you feel more empathetic and willing to compromise.

Empathy plays a huge role in these discussions. It's about really feeling what your partner is going through, which can help you respond in a more supportive and understanding way. This doesn't mean you'll always agree, but it ensures a strong current of love and respect, even during disagreements.

These conversations are about more than just solving issues—they're about connecting on a deeper level. They require courage, openness, and a better understanding of each other. Even though it's tough, having these talks with wisdom and a willingness to see each other's side can light up even the trickiest discussions about finances, intimacy, and parenting.

Creating a "Safe Space" for Open Dialogue

When trust grows, and understanding deepens, we create a safe space for our deepest thoughts and emotions. This safe space is free from the sting of judgment and retaliation, where being open helps strengthen our bonds. By valuing this safe space, our conversations become more than just talk; they turn into deep connections where respect, empathy, and acceptance guide everything we do.

Establishing Ground Rules

We start by setting some ground rules. These aren't just rules; they help us remember that we're here to respect each other, not to fight. These guidelines, which we create together, are all about being open and honest. They might include a rule about not interrupting, ensuring that when one person speaks, the other listens fully, showing respect for their words. Or they might stress keeping things confidential, ensuring that whatever is shared stays between us, safe and secure. These simple but essential rules help keep our conversations positive, steering us towards understanding and a stronger connection.

Encouraging Expression

In this space we've set up together, encouraging each other to open up becomes more about gentle nudges than considerable demands. It's about making each other feel safe enough to share the deeper parts of ourselves. When we invite each other to talk with simple, open-ended questions like, "How did that make you feel?" or "What are you hoping for?" it's not an interrogation. It's just a way to get those more profound thoughts and feelings out into the open, letting them breathe and grow.

Handling Emotional Responses

The strength of a relationship hinges on how both people manage their emotions. Emotions are part of who we are, not something to push away. These feelings shouldn't be ignored or brushed off but recognized and respected when they come up. It's about handling emotions carefully without necessarily buying into the whole story behind them. You acknowledge emotions by repeating to them what you hear without judgment, like saying, "You seem overwhelmed." This kind of validation lets emotions be felt and heard, which is critical to allowing them to pass or change.

Keeping a space open for honest talk is crucial. This means setting clear ground rules, inviting each other to share, and dealing with emotions in a way that builds trust and understanding. It's not about big dramatic gestures but the quiet moments you share, where real connection happens. In these moments, you go beyond just talking to connecting deeply through understanding and empathy. As you keep talking and sharing these quiet moments, your bond grows stronger, built on trust, respect, and a deep, shared openness.

The Role of Nonverbal Communication in Expressing Love

Nonverbal communication fills the gaps between what we say with a whole range of unspoken feelings, showing a lot without a single word. Our body language can express deep love and connection that words can't capture. Every gesture and look can show a wide range of emotions and thoughts. For instance, a genuine smile makes the person smiling light up and shows the person they're smiling at how much they mean to them. When you lean in during a conversation, it shows you're listening and caring about what's being said, valuing the other person's words.

Touch is another powerful way to show love, comfort, and care. Whether a reassuring pat on the back or a warm hug, every touch is loaded with meaning and can strengthen a bond by making the other person feel loved and cared for. However, it's crucial always to consider the context and ensure everyone's comfortable with physical touch to ensure these actions are respectful and welcomed.

Picking up on nonverbal cues requires a sharp intuition because our body language often subtly reflects our feelings more than words. Noticing a slight change in someone's posture or facial expression can tell much about their mood or feelings. Reacting correctly to these cues means combining empathy with the right action—maybe a nod, a touch, or a supportive glance, which can all acknowledge the other person's feelings without saying it aloud.

Nonverbal communication is a powerful relationship tool, helping us connect beyond words. By paying close attention to these silent signals and responding thoughtfully, relationships can grow stronger and be filled with understanding and empathy, making the most of all those meaningful moments without a word being spoken.

Maintaining Intimacy and Passion

Keeping the spark alive is crucial but challenging due to routine and obligations. It's about creating special moments and experiences, not just letting time pass. Setting up regular date nights shows we're invested in each other's happiness. These aren't just breaks from daily life but chances to focus solely on each other, whether that's dinner out or just chilling under the stars.

Beyond date nights, integrating quality time into everyday life is key. It could be sharing a laugh over morning coffee, holding hands, or just enjoying a quiet moment together. These small interactions build a deeper connection, filling everyday life with shared joys and comfort.

It's also fun to shake things up by trying new things together, like taking a dance class or cooking a new dish, even if it ends in a food fight. These adventures can bring excitement and a sense of teamwork into the relationship, creating memories and showing how you can adapt and enjoy new experiences together.

Open communication about your desires and what you expect from each other is also vital. This talk can be tough—sharing your wants and needs takes guts. But this openness is the safety net that makes these conversations possible, helping to deepen trust and understanding. Discussing your needs and listening to each other creates a partnership that fulfills your dreams.

Ultimately, it's about cherishing the big adventures and the quiet, everyday moments. You keep the relationship exciting and strong by making time for dates, enjoying simple daily interactions, and trying new things together. It's about moving forward together, always remembering to nurture the connection that brought you together in the first place.

Preventing Resentment in Your Relationship

When resentment builds up, it can chill the warmth of a marriage, leaving it feeling pretty cold. It's like not caring for a garden—before you know it, all those weeds of old grudges and unspoken issues can choke out the love and companionship that should be growing. To keep this from happening, you've got to put in daily effort, keeping the lines of communication open and showing each other appreciation.

Start with regular relationship check-ins. Think of it as the time to nurture your relationship, where you can talk, reflect, and listen to each other without the noise of everyday life getting in the way. It's your chance to air out any issues, share what's been good, and plan for what's ahead. This helps keep you both on the same page and nip problems in the bud before they grow.

Remember to show appreciation, too. It's simple but powerful and keeps the relationship from getting neglected. A little "thank you" here, a "good job" there—these moments of gratitude make a big difference. They remind you both why you're doing this together.

Tackling problems before they turn into resentment takes guts. It means speaking up about what's bothering you, being open about your feelings, and having those tough conversations. But these aren't just complaints; they're opportunities to understand each other better, make adjustments, and grow stronger together. It's about facing these issues together, not letting them build up.

Managing a marriage, especially a remarriage, involves a lot of upkeep. Both partners must be committed to checking in, expressing gratitude, and confronting issues early on. This ongoing effort helps keep the relationship fresh and resilient, ensuring it thrives.

As we wrap up, it's clear that preventing resentment is more than avoiding arguments. It's about creating a dynamic where discovery, renewal, and deep companionship can flourish. By sticking to these practices, you can ensure your relationship survives and thrives, lighting up your lives with joy and mutual support.

SIX

Financial Harmony and Creating a New Blend

M oney matters a lot, and in a remarriage, handling it together becomes super important. You've got to blend your different ways of dealing with finances into one smooth operation. It's a bit tricky and requires both of you to be flexible and attentive. We will look at how you can merge finances with your partner. Sure, it might be tough at times, but it's also a great chance to create a solid financial future that keeps you both feeling secure and lets you have independence.

Merging Finances: A Roadmap for Couples

In remarriages, you need a clear financial plan that both of you agree on. It's all about creating a plan that respects your dreams, responsibilities, and worries, not just about who pays the bills or saves for a rainy day. When you merge finances, it's a careful balance between maintaining your independence and working towards common goals.

Joint vs. Separate Accounts

Deciding whether to go for joint or separate bank accounts is a big remarriage decision. Joint accounts can show you're in this together, making managing your budget and everyday expenses easier. They symbolize a commitment to shared financial goals and responsibilities, sticking to the "what's mine is yours" vibe. On the flip side, having separate accounts lets each person handle their own money how they see fit, which can be great for maintaining financial independence. This is especially handy in remarriages, where you might want to manage your expenses or have personal financial commitments, like child support or paying off old debts.

A mix of both often works best. You can have a joint account that takes care of household costs like the mortgage, utilities, and shared savings goals, while separate accounts cover personal spending and savings. This setup allows for teamwork on common expenses while respecting each person's financial independence.

Setting Financial Goals

Aligning your financial goals means sitting down together and mapping out what you want from your money. Maybe it's saving up for a big vacation, putting money away for your kid's college fund, or planning retirement. These goals act as guides for your spending and saving. It all starts with an honest talk about what's important to you both, what you're worried about, and what you hope to achieve. Then, you break these goals down into when you want to hit them: short-term (within a year), medium-term (one to five years), and long-term (beyond five years).

Checking in on these goals regularly is key to keeping everything on track. This helps ensure they make sense for your life together, especially as things change inside and outside your relationship.

Budgeting as a Team

A budget is essential, but it's more than keeping track of what's coming in and going out. It's about building a framework of support and working towards common goals. You start by being open about your financial situation—lay out your income, expenses, debts, and assets. From there, you can shape a budget that reflects what you aim to achieve together, ensuring your money goes where it needs to.

The best way to handle this as a team is to break your expenses into categories. You've got your must-haves, like rent and groceries; your obligations, like debts or child support payments; and your wants, including fun money and savings. This way, you can see where your money's going, figure out where to save, and make space for shared dreams and personal wishes.

Visual Element: Financial Goals Worksheet

You can use a worksheet to set and track your financial goals. It'll have spots for the goal's name, its importance (high, medium, or low), when you want to hit it, the estimated cost, and how you're doing so far. This tool allows couples to lay out their financial dreams together and figure out how to achieve them during their money talks.

Merging finances isn't just about sorting out who pays for what; it's a chance to strengthen your partnership. You get to share your goals, support each other, and have real talks about money. It's all about building a life together where both partners' efforts unite seamlessly, showcasing unity and individuality. Deciding whether to mix your money or keep it separate, setting joint financial goals, and making a budget can all help you craft a financial future that fits your shared life perfectly.

Addressing Debt: Strategies for a Clean Financial Slate

Dealing with debt in a remarriage isn't just about the money; it's a major stressor that can mess with the peace of your relationship. If you ignore it, it can lead to secrets, distrust, and a lot of tension. So, managing debt is crucial—not just for your bank account but for keeping your relationship healthy and strong. It's important to recognize how stressful debt can be and carefully plan how to get rid of it together.

Full Disclosure

Kicking things off with total honesty about your debts isn't just sharing numbers; it's about showing trust and opening up in your relationship. It's not about admitting defeat—it's about wanting to tackle everything together. When you lay it all out there—the credit card debts, loans, whatever baggage from before—it sets you both up to tackle these issues as a team. Being open about finances is not just a practical step; it's about building a foundation of trust and starting on a path to financial and emotional stability.

Debt Repayment Plans

Once you've laid out all your debts, crafting a repayment plan is the next step. This isn't a one-size-fits-all solution but a personalized strategy considering your financial situation and how ready you feel to tackle it. You might knock out the smaller debts using the snowball method or go after the ones with the highest interest first with the avalanche method. Remember, this plan can change. It's flexible and meant to adapt to your financial ups and downs and future goals.

Tackling this plan means you must be all in, understanding and valuing each other's contributions to clearing the debt. It's about finding the right balance—staying ambitious about wiping out debts while maintaining a lifestyle that keeps you both happy and stress-free. You might find it helpful to consolidate your debts for a better interest rate or renegotiate payment terms with your creditors. The best strategy will be one that you're both comfortable with and allows for adjustments along the way.

Impact on Financial Goals

Managing debt while focusing on your bigger financial goals is like balancing short-term challenges with your long-term dreams. It's not just about getting rid of debt; it's about how clearing that debt fits into your shared plans, like saving up for a house, planning for retirement, or setting aside money for the kids' education. You must understand how these immediate pressures mesh with your future aspirations.

As you work through this, you might discover that knocking out debt speeds up your overall financial progress, freeing up more cash for saving and investing sooner. Or, you might decide on a steadier debt repayment plan that allows you to keep contributing to your savings, avoiding too much financial stress. In remarriage, managing finances is all about flexibility because handling debt and pursuing your dreams should go hand in hand, not compete against each other.

In doing this, how you handle debt reflects how you handle your marriage: openness, support for each other, and the flexibility to adapt. By tackling debt together, you're not just dealing with numbers but reinforcing your partnership. It's about moving together through life's ups and downs, handling every challenge as a team. This journey is more than just about budgets or spreadsheets; it's about building a life together, step by step.

Planning for the Future: Retirement, Education and Savings

When you remarry, planning for the future is more than just being smart with your money—it's about bringing your dreams together and setting shared goals. It's a careful balancing act, managing resources, figuring out what's most important, and setting timelines that respect your independence and life together.

Retirement Planning: Harmonizing Visions

Planning for retirement isn't just about the money—it's about blending your past experiences, current life, and future dreams. This task means you have to get on the same page about what you want your retirement to look like. It's more than just crunching numbers; it's about understanding each other's hopes, fears, and what you're both willing to compromise on.

You'll need to look at existing retirement accounts, any pension benefits you might have, and what it means to combine these resources. Understanding how this will work legally and tax-wise is essential to ensure your plans support your financial goals while fitting into the broader rules of estate laws and retirement regulations. This planning ensures you both can enjoy your later years as you envisioned.

Keeping an open line of communication is vital. Regular talks about your retirement dreams, worries, and expectations are crucial. Financial planning tools and retirement calculators can help make sense of the numbers. But at the core of retirement planning is your ability to work through emotional challenges together, ensuring your financial strategies reflect your shared visions for the future.

Education Savings: A Unified Front

Planning for the kids' education, whether from previous or current relationships, adds a twist to your financial planning when you're remarried. But tackling this challenge isn't just about money—it's a chance to strengthen your family ties and show your kids you're invested in their futures.

You need to be smart about dividing your resources, ensuring you meet each child's educational needs without messing up your family's finances or plans. Tax-advantaged savings accounts like 529 plans or Coverdell Education Savings Accounts can help significantly. These accounts are designed to boost your savings for your kids' education costs, tailored to each child's needs.

It's crucial to weave these education savings into your overall financial plan. This means balancing how much you put into these education accounts with how much you need to save for retirement or pay off debts. By handling it this way, you reinforce that you value everyone's dreams and are working to make them possible. It's about ensuring your financial plan covers everyone's goals and strengthening your family unit.

Emergency Fund: The Safety Net

Setting up an emergency fund is wise for couples serious about securing their future together. This fund is like a safety net, ready to catch you if sudden expenses hit—whether that's a medical issue, losing a job, or needing to fix something big at home.

Starting this fund means regularly setting aside a chunk of your family's income in an emergency savings account. How much you stash away depends on how stable your jobs are, your health, and what safety nets you have, like insurance. Having enough to cover three to six months of living expenses is a good idea.

But an emergency fund is more than just intelligent money management. It's a clear sign of how much you care for each other. It shows you're committed to looking after your shared life, no matter what surprises come. With this fund in place, you can chase your long-term dreams without worrying too much because you know you have a backup plan for those just-in-case moments.

Navigating Child Support and Alimony With Transparency

Handling child support and alimony can get complicated when past financial commitments are combined with current ones. Being transparent and open in your communication is vital. It's super important for building trust in your new family setup. By discussing things openly, couples can respect their past responsibilities while caring for their new relationship.

Budgeting for Obligations

The budgeting process for child support and alimony requires careful planning and foresight. It's crucial to allocate every dollar carefully so the household can meet its legal obligations while supporting its current and future needs. These obligations are fixed expenses central to your family's financial structure. By treating child support and alimony as essential parts of the budget you help strengthen and stabilize your family's financial health. Incorporating these payments into your financial planning can help reduce stress and create a healthier environment for everyone.

Legal Adjustments

When your financial situation changes unexpectedly, adjusting child support or alimony payments should be handled carefully. This means looking at your family's new financial landscape and talking to a lawyer about updating those payments to match your current situation. Being open with your partner and anyone affected by these changes is important. By dealing with these adjustments transparently, you can ensure that everyone's financial contributions stay fair and adapt to changes like a new job, a change in income, or other significant life events. Keeping everyone in the loop and being honest about your situation helps maintain trust and keeps everything above board in your relationship.

Impact on New Family Dynamics

The new family dynamic depends on stability, trust, and understanding in every remarriage. Handling child support and alimony openly is key to keeping this dynamic healthy. It shows a commitment to fairness and helps prevent bitterness or confusion from financial ties to past relationships. This openness can turn a tension point into a chance for growth, showing that everyone is on the same page and values the whole family's well-being. This approach helps strengthen the family's bonds, creating an environment where everyone feels valued and secure, no matter where they fit in the blended family structure.

Remarriage requires clear communication, especially about financial matters like child support and alimony. You've got to be ready to adjust to changes in financial situations and understand how these obligations affect the family dynamic. By handling these matters openly, couples can ensure their relationship properly blends past, present, and future financial responsibilities, meets their obligations and strengthens the foundation of their new family, setting them up for a stable, understanding, and fulfilling future together.

Insurance and Estate Planning

As blended families become more complicated, ensuring the right insurance and estate planning becomes super important. It's not just another thing to check off your marriage to-do list; it's about protecting everyone in your family from life's unexpected turns. This planning helps you look after your family's future, not just the day-to-day. It's about leaving a lasting legacy and covering all your bases.

Life Insurance Considerations

Getting the right life insurance is crucial because it ensures your family is financially secure if something unexpected happens to you. It isn't just about picking any policy; it's about choosing one that fits what your family needs, wants, and can afford—whether it's a whole-life policy that lasts your entire life and builds cash value or term life, which covers you for a certain period.

You must consider your debt, future expenses, and the lifestyle you hope to maintain. It's essential to ensure that a spouse who cares for kids from previous relationships can handle the situation. Getting life insurance is a significant move—it's not just about the money; it's a way to show you care about your family's future even when you're not around.

Estate Planning Complexities

Estate planning in a blended family is tricky because you're juggling past commitments and future promises. You've got to ensure that how you leave your assets reflects what both partners want and honors their legacy. Blended families face unique challenges like navigating through legal rules, handling emotional factors, and dealing with their complex structure.

Hiring a lawyer helps make sense of the tricky parts of wills, trusts, and estates. They're experts in determining what the laws say and assisting couples in creating estate plans that capture their wishes. This includes making clear, legally sound documents that detail who gets what, who will take care of the kids, and who makes decisions if you can't.

Guardianship and Inheritance

Guardianship and inheritance are big deals when planning an estate in a blended family. These decisions pack much emotional punch and require deeper thought and understanding.

Choosing a guardian for your kids can be challenging. You have to think about who shares your values, how they approach parenting, and the emotional connection they have with your kids. It's all about ensuring your kids are loved and cared for if you're not around. When it comes to passing down your stuff, you've got to be thoughtful and make sure you respect the financial legacy you want to leave for each kid, considering all the stepfamily dynamics.

Trusts are a standard tool here. They let you set aside money for things like your kids' education or help them out as they grow up, ensuring your money is used exactly how you want. Trusts are great in blended families because they allow you to tailor things just right, reflecting your juggling complex relationships and responsibilities.

Getting estate planning right in a blended family means thinking long-term and committing to caring for your family correctly. It's not just about money—it's about showing love and responsibility, protecting your family's future and honoring your wishes. With careful planning, clear communication, and some legal help, you can ensure your family is set up right for whatever comes their way.

Budgeting Together: Aligning Your Financial Goals

Making a budget isn't just about crunching numbers. It's really about blending your past experiences and future hopes into a plan that works for both of you. This task is more than just filling out spreadsheets; it's about showing how committed you are to building a harmonious life together. As you assemble a budget, you get a real sense of what matters to each other, from your biggest worries to your wildest dreams.

Crafting a Joint Budget: A Symphony of Numbers

Setting up a joint budget is about precision and understanding each other. Start by laying all your cards on the table—how much you earn, what you owe, and your regular expenses. But this isn't just about numbers; it's about building trust. Openly sharing financial details should bring you closer, not create stress.

With all the info out, you can create a budget that fits boring and fun stuff. You figure out how much you need for the essentials and set aside some cash to enjoy life. This budgeting process isn't just practical; it's also about making room for each other's dreams. Through honest communication and respect, you work on a financial plan that supports your life together, balancing day-to-day needs with your more significant hopes for the future.

Prioritizing Expenses: A Deliberate Choice

Navigating life's expenses together means more than just crunching numbers; it's about understanding what matters to both of you. Your long-term plans and immediate needs help you decide where to focus your money without having to cut corners for the sake of saving; it's about spending in ways that bring you closer to your shared dreams, like saving for a future home, investing wisely, or knocking out debts.

When you make these decisions together, what might feel like sacrifices become intelligent choices for a better future. Balancing what you both need and want from life makes your budget more than just a spreadsheet—it becomes a tool that adapts and grows with your relationship. This way, your budget doesn't just tell you where your money's going. It supports your journey together, reflecting your goals and the life you're building.

Regular Budget Reviews: Navigating Change

The financial side of a remarriage is constantly changing, just like life itself. An annual budget review is crucial—it's like your personal check-in point that lets you reassess your goals, celebrate what you've achieved, and tweak your plans as needed. This budget review isn't just a routine task; it's a critical moment for connection. It's a chance for both of you to look back at the year, recognize what you've accomplished, and face any new challenges together.

This review isn't about pointing fingers or finding faults. It's about working together to adapt to whatever life throws your way. Changes in income, unexpected bills, or achieving a financial goal—these reviews are an honest conversation about where you are and where you want to be. They ensure your budget reflects your current situation and your plans for the future.

By doing these check-ins regularly, you keep your budget aligned with your life's rhythm. It's about staying proactive and adaptable, navigating through remarriage with a clear map. Budgeting becomes about managing money and continuing to build your relationship. It's a way to show love and reaffirm your commitment to a future that respects your needs and dreams. By working together on your budget, setting priorities, and staying on top of regular reviews, you turn the financial challenges of remarriage into chances for growth, understanding, and a stronger bond.

The Importance of Financial Independence

Financial independence isn't about driving a wedge between partners. Instead, it's crucial for keeping things smooth and healthy. It's all about finding the right balance between being your own person and part of a team. Having your own money means you can maintain your sense of self and personal space within the marriage, which helps strengthen the relationship. This independence allows you to chase your dreams together without losing sight of your goals and needs.

Personal Spending Money

Setting aside personal spending money in the budget shows respect for each partner's individuality and their need to express themselves. This financial freedom isn't about giving each other an allowance; it's about acknowledging that both of you should have the space to explore personal interests or enjoy a bit of independence. Spending on yourself or your hobbies isn't a breach of trust—it adds layers of respect, trust, and satisfaction to your relationship, making it more robust because you both feel valued.

Individual Investments

Having your investments is smart for keeping your family financially secure because it lets you dive into the financial world on your terms and boosts your family's financial health. Whether it's stocks, retirement accounts, or real estate, these investments are not just about money—they represent your interests, how much risk you're comfortable with, and your personal growth. Investing on your own can make you feel more empowered and bring new insights and experiences into your relationship, which adds to its richness.

At the same time, it's crucial to keep the lines of communication open and maintain mutual respect as you balance these personal investments with your joint financial goals. Doing this means being open to discussing priorities and supporting each other's financial endeavors, ensuring these individual pursuits complement rather than clash with your shared plans. As you and your relationship grow and change, finding the right balance between personal and joint financial activities can help ensure everyone feels secure and valued.

Balancing Independence With Unity

In a healthy remarriage, it's all about striking the right balance between having financial independence and working together as a team. This balance respects each partner's individuality, recognizing that the union's strength comes from both people bringing their unique selves to the table. Getting this right involves a lot of open communication, mutual respect, and shared values.

Couples often have regular financial meetings to discuss and celebrate their individual and shared goals. It's crucial to set clear financial boundaries and make agreements that respect each partner's need for financial autonomy while still looking out for the family's finances. Creating a transparent environment for making personal and shared financial decisions builds trust and teamwork, which are essential for a successful remarriage.

This setup allows both partners to feel supported in their financial activities and committed to their joint financial goals. Personal growth and shared progress go hand in hand, enhancing the other. In a remarriage, financial independence doesn't pull partners apart;

instead, it adds strength, diversity, and resilience, enriching the relationship.

Financial independence is vital in a remarriage, where past experiences play into present plans. By smartly managing personal spending money, exploring individual investments, and finding the right balance between personal and joint finances, couples can honor the complexities of their blended lives. This approach respects each partner's autonomy and strengthens their bond, enabling both to thrive individually and as a couple, united by common goals and enriched by their pursuits.

Legal Implications of Financial Decisions in Remarriage

Considering the legal side when remarrying and blending lives and finances is essential because it isn't just about mixing money; it's about understanding the laws that affect how you can merge your finances. Navigating this can bring you closer together or cause issues, so you must handle it carefully.

Within the rules and agreements the law sets out, couples can find what they need to build a future that looks out for both partners, getting a good grasp on these legal guidelines and using them to protect everyone's interests as they come together.

Prenuptial Agreements

Prenuptial agreements are like setting the ground rules before you get married. They clear up how you'll handle money and divide assets if things don't work out. Even though some might think this looks like you're betting against the marriage, it's about making things crystal clear from the start. Crafting these agreements is a delicate balance. You've got to protect each person while still honoring the partnership, which means having open and honest talks where you recognize what each of you brings to the table and where you might be vulnerable. A well-done prenup creates a safe space, ensuring that individual and joint finances are sorted out. This clarity allows your relationship to grow without any financial uncertainties.

Name Changes and Credit

Changing your last name after getting remarried can feel like a fresh start, but it also means dealing with some paperwork headaches. This change touches everything from your bank accounts to your credit score. You'll need to update your name with credit card companies, banks, and credit bureaus to ensure your financial identity isn't lost in the shuffle. It might seem straightforward, but it's a bit of a chore. This is important because your credit can affect everything from taking out loans to passing identity checks. You must handle this change carefully to ensure it doesn't jeopardize your new marriage's financial situation.

Marital Property Laws

When couples blend their lives and assets in remarriage, they have to navigate a complex set of laws that influence how assets are split and categorized, depending on where they live. Couples must get a grip on these rules to make smart financial choices about personal vs. marital property. In places with community property laws, anything you gain during the marriage is owned together, which means you need to think carefully about how you manage and acquire assets. On the other hand, states with common law systems pose challenges and opportunities by differentiating between individual and shared assets.

Leveraging these laws means adjusting your financial habits to fit legal requirements, which includes deciding how future assets are classified, dealing with debts before marriage, and managing inheritances to ensure your asset management is legal and matches your mutual goals.

In this complex legal and personal landscape, the legal side of financial decisions in remarriage is foundational for building your future together. It demands careful attention, thorough understanding, and teamwork. By strategically planning everything from prenups to handling changes in names and credit and navigating property laws, you can set up a framework that supports legal needs and your relationship goals. This approach helps make financial decisions solid pillars for stability and growth in your remarried life.

Financial Conflict Resolution: Finding Common Ground

It's not just a sign of trouble when old financial issues reappear. Instead, it's a chance to get on the same page and strengthen the relationship. These financial conflicts often stem from blending past financial habits with new commitments and dealing with them requires more than basic problem-solving. It's about reaching a compromise and respecting each other's backgrounds and values. This process involves using solid communication tactics that help both partners agree. Bringing in a professional can make a big difference, helping clear up confusion and point the way forward.

Understanding Differing Values

Financial disagreements are more than just about the numbers—they're about what those numbers mean based on our backgrounds, past experiences with money, and deep-seated beliefs about spending, saving, and sharing it. Recognizing and respecting these differences is the first step when sorting out finances with your partner. It's crucial to listen to each other's money stories and see these differences as chances to bring diverse perspectives into your financial plans, not as roadblocks. This approach can transform financial decisions from potential arguments into opportunities to connect different pasts with a shared vision for the future.

Communication Strategies

Handling financial disagreements is about talking with empathy and keeping the conversation positive. You want to ensure you focus on "we" when you talk money, highlighting how each decision impacts your shared plans, not just personal complaints. Turning potentially tough talks into team efforts starts by framing these discussions around your shared goals. Using "I feel" statements helps shift the focus from pointing fingers to sharing personal feelings, which opens the door to understanding each other better without getting defensive.

Having these chats in a calm, neutral place away from daily distractions ensures the conversation gets the serious attention it deserves. Setting up a space like this makes it easier for everyone to be honest and open, keeping the focus on solutions that work best for both of you. Also, having a clear agenda with specific topics and objectives can help keep the discussion on track, steering clear of the side issues that complicate money talks.

Professional Financial Advice

Sometimes, to fix money issues, you need help from experts. That's where a financial advisor or counselor comes in handy. They can clear up any confusion about finances with their expertise and offer a neutral point of view that can help both partners understand each other better. These pros can guide the conversation, ask the right questions, and point out solutions you might not have considered because you're too close to the problem or need all the info.

Getting professional advice shows you're serious about making your relationship work long-term and you're open to using outside resources to strengthen your bond. Whether it's about combining assets, sorting out debts, or planning for big future goals, a financial pro can take the stress out of not knowing what to do, making money management a solid part of your relationship rather than a constant battle.

Tackling financial conflicts together is not just a challenge; it's an opportunity. It lets couples better understand each other's financial viewpoints, work out strategies that respect both sides and build a strong relationship in all areas. By respecting each other's views, using intelligent communication strategies, and sometimes calling in a pro, you can handle financial disagreements in a way that strengthens your bond. Instead of causing fights, these challenges can help you grow together, building a relationship founded on mutual respect, understanding, and shared goals. With this approach, money problems can help you build a more harmonious and satisfying life together.

Celebrating Financial Milestones Together

When you're remarried, hitting financial milestones isn't just a sign of progress; it's a big deal that celebrates what you've achieved and the dreams you still want to chase. Celebrating these moments strengthens your marriage by bringing fresh energy and a sense of achievement. It's about more than just patting yourselves on the back —it's a way to reinforce the resilience, commitment, and teamwork that define your journey together.

Defining Milestones: Crafting Markers of Success

The first thing you need to do when celebrating financial wins in a remarriage is to figure out what counts as a milestone for you and your partner, which means more than just making a list of goals. You must dig into what matters to both of you and agree on which achievements you want to celebrate. It could be anything from paying off a significant debt, hitting a savings goal, or reaching an investment milestone. These are important because they show what you've accomplished together and highlight each partner's contributions to your financial well-being.

Talking about and defining these milestones is an ongoing thing that adapts as your financial life and priorities change. It's about diving deep and having honest conversations, which gets you both on the same page and strengthens your bond around money. This approach ensures you celebrate your joint successes and individual financial strides.

Celebration Ideas: Honoring Achievement Without Undermining Goals

Chatting about your financial milestones is excellent for setting up a celebration, acknowledging your hard work and motivating you toward your shared financial goals. But keeping these celebrations in line with your financial plan is critical. Go for creative, meaningful ways to celebrate that make sure your budget is reasonable.

You have many options for celebrating, depending on what you both enjoy and the milestone you've reached. Have a special dinner where you can talk about your financial journey and what you're aiming for next. Or, you could go for a small, thoughtful gift that symbolizes your achievements or use some extra cash for a shared experience or a future project. These celebrations can make your achievements feel special without derailing your financial plans.

Reflecting on Progress: Fueling Future Aspirations

Celebrating financial milestones is about taking a moment to reflect. It's not just about reviewing what you've accomplished but also digging into the lessons you learned along the way, the obstacles you overcame, and how you've grown. It's a time to acknowledge the hard work, resilience, and support that got you to this point, and it reinforces your commitment to your shared financial goals and plans as a couple.

This reflection moment also sparks future ideas, motivating you to set new goals and tweak your financial plans. Achieving one goal sets you up for the next, creating a cycle of goal-setting, achieving, and celebrating that keeps pushing both of you toward your vision of financial harmony.

So, celebrating these milestones is more than just a pat on the back— it's a vital part of your financial strategy as a couple. It strengthens your bond, keeps you focused on your financial goals and fosters a culture of appreciation and support. It shows you how far you've come and points the way forward, spotlighting what you can achieve together. From these celebrations to discussions on maintaining individual identities within your marriage, the key lessons are collaboration, resilience, and shared commitment—foundations for financial success and a strong, lasting partnership.

SEVEN

Building a Future With Shared Dreams and Goals

Imagine a couple sitting at their kitchen table littered with remnants of breakfast, the morning sun casting a soft glow around them. Amid the mundane chaos of their daily lives, they carve out this moment to dream—to share, listen, and weave together aspirations that span from the immediate to the distant future. In these seemingly ordinary yet profoundly significant moments, the foundation for a unified direction in marriage is laid. Shared dreams and goals are not just lofty ideals but the threads that bind two people together, turning individual hopes into a collective journey.

The Power of Shared Dreams and Goals

Aligning shared dreams and goals is about building a shared story where both partners feel their aspirations are seen and valued. This shared vision guides your choices, actions, and compromises, ensuring everything points toward your desired future. It's like building a bridge between two lives, and the success of that bridge relies on how clear and strong your shared vision is.

Vision Creation

Think about making a vision board, a physical display of your shared dreams and goals. Fill it with images, quotes, and symbols that remind you of where you want to go together. This isn't just a fun, creative project; it's a powerful way to keep your dreams right before you, making them real and touchable. Whether it's picturing a cozy house in the countryside, a life full of travel and excitement, or a quiet life focused on giving back, this board stands as a visible commitment to those shared dreams.

Unity and Motivation

This shared vision is beneficial when times get tough, reminding you why you're in this together. It acts like a guide, keeping you on track when things get rocky. Whenever you face challenges, just looking at your vision board—with all the images and words you both chose—can boost your motivation and remind you of the larger goals and reasons you started this journey together.

Collaborative Visioning

To keep your shared vision alive, consider having regular "dream sessions." These aren't just regular chats but special times to share your most significant dreams without worrying about the here and now. It's a chance to ask, "What if?" and "Why not?" without getting bogged down by practical details. Treat these sessions like essential meetings because you're planning your future together. Use this time to cheer each other on, expand on each other's ideas, and let the excitement about what you could achieve keep your enthusiasm burning.

Visual Element: Vision Board Template

Using a template can help when you're trying to visualize your future together. This handy tool lets you organize images, quotes, and symbols that reflect what you both want out of life. You can break it down into your home, travel plans, careers, family, hobbies, and personal development. Every time you add something to the board, you're not just making a collage of your dreams but reinforcing your commitment to making them happen.

Creating this shared vision is super personal. It's like saying to each other, "I see our future with you, and I want you in it." It's about understanding that life might not stick to your plan, but having a shared direction can keep your bond strong against challenges and make victories even sweeter. This vision board becomes the backdrop of your life story together, one that you both write one dream at a time.

Blending Your Values and Traditions

In remarriage, you get to blend two different values and traditions into one. It's more than just making room for each other's pasts; it's about building something new together. You're not compromising but creating a new shared identity that respects your background. Together, you create a unique mix of values and traditions that reflects the complexity and beauty of your partnership. This isn't just mixing things; it's about making something beautiful and new that stands for both of you.

Respect and Inclusion

Respect is key in making a marriage work, especially when blending different values and traditions. It means listening to each other, keeping an open heart, and trying to see things from your partner's perspective. Every tradition and value that each partner brings to the table is a big part of who they are, shaped by their past experiences and the legacy of their families. By honoring these in your new family culture, you show respect for where your partner comes from, recognize their worth, and accept their past. This isn't just about getting along; it's about growing together and making your life richer with the diversity of each other's backgrounds.

Negotiating Differences

Navigating the differences in values and traditions when blending lives is like steering a boat through merging waters. It takes skill to manage where past, present, individual, and shared elements meet. The key is open dialogue, where listening matters as much as speaking. The goal isn't to water down or overshadow each other's backgrounds but to understand and find common ground. This doesn't mean ignoring your differences; instead, it celebrates them as strengths that enrich your relationship. Some values may be non-negotiable and deeply tied to who you are, while others might be more flexible ready to mix and evolve. Through this process of compromise and adjustment, you create a new set of shared values and traditions that reflect both of your identities yet form a unique bond.

Creating New Traditions

Creating new traditions is really about using your imagination together. It's about shaping "what could be" and solidifying who you are as a team. These traditions grow from blending your pasts and become the markers for celebrating time passing, achievements, and even offering comfort during tough times. They turn holidays, birthdays, and anniversaries into meaningful moments of continuity and belonging.

Creating new traditions is also about leaving a legacy for any kids you might be raising together, bringing pieces of your journey into their futures. Whether blending old traditions into something new or creating completely fresh rituals, it's all about crafting a shared story. This process requires you to consider the values, moments, and memories you want to celebrate regularly.

By doing this, you respect and include each other's backgrounds, using your differences as strengths rather than obstacles. It's a journey of co-creation, making a culture that's uniquely yours and strengthens your bond. It's not just about overcoming challenges but about embracing the chance to build something that honors both your histories and the future you're aiming for together. This work isn't just about compromise; it's a profound expression of your commitment to each other and the life you're building.

Establishing New Family Norms and Cultures

Creating new family norms ensures everyone in your blended family feels at home. It's not just about merging old habits and traditions; it's about shaping a space where everyone can thrive and feel accepted. This involves establishing rules that reflect what your family is about while keeping things flexible enough to change as life evolves. It's a collaborative journey where the entire family works together to figure out how to blend their lives in ways that work for everyone.

Norm Setting

Setting family norms is all about balancing everyone's needs while creating a vibe that everyone's on the same team. Think of it like working with clay—everyone gets their hands dirty shaping these rules, influenced by what everyone thinks, feels, and hopes for. This way, everyone feels they have a stake in the game, which builds respect and understanding.

Kicking off this process means pulling everyone together for family meetings. These aren't stiff, formal affairs but warm get-togethers where everyone gets a say. You'll talk about the everyday stuff like chores, bedtime routines, house rules and the more significant things like how you support each other emotionally, handle disagreements and make decisions together. From these talks, you'll start to see a set of norms take shape, sort of a living guide that helps steer the family's daily life, ensuring there's enough give in the rules to meet everyone's changing needs.

Cultural Blend

Mixing different cultural backgrounds creates a vibrant setting for establishing new family norms and cultures. Far from watering down individual heritages, this blend enriches the family's collective identity, creating a mosaic that celebrates diversity. Each cultural element—a holiday celebration, a favorite dish, or a unique way of speaking—adds color and texture to the family's shared experiences.

Engaging with and being curious about each other's backgrounds are vital to navigating this blend. Imagine having cooking nights where everyone prepares dishes from their own cultures or language days where everyone shares phrases and stories from their heritage. Celebrating different holidays together can also become a unique family tradition. These aren't just fun activities but important rituals that help everyone feel included and valued. Through these shared experiences, the family builds a unique culture that respects everyone's past while creating a new, unified future.

Flexibility and Evolution

When creating new family norms and cultures, it is important to remember that they can change and adapt over time. This flexibility helps the family adjust to new situations and grow together, whether due to changes in who's in the family, what people want out of life, or just the passing of time.

To make this work, families must continue talking to each other openly, considering how things are going, and being willing to tweak or change their norms based on new experiences. Regular family meetings can determine if the current norms still fit or if new ones are needed. Doing this together, with everyone's input, helps the family stay strong and on the same page.

This ability to adapt shows a family's strength and capacity to stick together through life's highs and lows. Creating these norms is not just about setting rules or mixing traditions; it's about building a culture of respect and growth that reflects the family's ongoing journey.

Establishing these norms is crucial in cases like remarriage, where families blend. It involves respecting each person's background while building a shared way of life. This process helps everyone get along and lays a foundation for a family legacy that values unity and collective growth, celebrating the complex journey they share.

Setting Goals: Short-Term Wins and Long-Term Visions

It's beneficial for couples to set both short-term and long-term goals. Doing this keeps me feeling purposeful, and the future looks hopeful. By having these goals, couples can keep moving forward and stay focused, even as things in their relationship change over time. Setting these goals helps them navigate the challenges of blending their lives, making sure they're always making progress, whether it's big or small steps.

Goal Categorization

It helps to sort your goals into three categories: personal, marital, and family-oriented. This helps keep everything balanced, ensuring you're paying attention to what each partner wants, what the relationship needs, and what the whole family needs to work well together.

This setup does more than just organize things; it's about finding a balance. Personal goals focus on growth, like getting ahead at work or improving your health. Marital goals are about strengthening the relationship, like building a deeper emotional connection or getting your finances on track. Family-oriented goals look at the bigger picture, like creating a solid family bond or planning fun trips together.

By splitting goals up this way, you can better handle the ins and outs of a blended family, making sure everyone grows together, individually and as a unit.

Achievable Milestones

Setting realistic short-term goals is critical to keeping up momentum and staying motivated. These goals are like checkpoints showing you're progressing toward your bigger dreams. They're the small wins that keep you moving forward, proving that you and your partner are doing the work and sticking to your commitments.

Making these goals means looking at what you can realistically achieve right now, considering what's possible within your current situation. It's all about recognizing and celebrating each small victory, knowing that these steps are building up to something bigger. For example, a short-term goal could be putting away a little money for a vacation you're dreaming about or spending a few hours each week on a hobby you both enjoy. These small but meaningful goals help weave your relationship together, giving you something to look forward to and a sense of achievement.

Review and Adjust

Remarriage is all about adapting to change. It's essential for couples to regularly check and adjust their goals to make sure they're still on track with their shared vision. This means sitting down together, looking at how far they've come, and tweaking their plans to fit better their current situation and what they hope to achieve together. Whether done monthly or quarterly, these reviews allow couples to pause, reassess, and recommit to their journey together.

Setting personal, marital, and family goals helps balance individual needs with collective aims. By creating achievable milestones, couples experience the satisfaction of making progress. Regularly reviewing and adjusting these goals gives them the flexibility to handle the changing dynamics of their relationship, keeping their shared vision relevant and aligned with their lives. This careful planning helps couples build a future where every success marks their commitment to each other and their family's resilience and unity.

Navigating Differences: When Visions Collide

When two people come together, they face a point where their goals might only sometimes align perfectly, which can be tough. However, this isn't a battlefield; it's a chance for both partners to grow and transform together. Handling these differences with understanding and compromise is crucial. It's not just about getting past hurdles;

it's an opportunity to strengthen the relationship and enrich it beyond just the individual contributions.

Resolving conflicts over different visions and goals is key to a smooth remarriage. This process involves more than just negotiating; it requires genuine empathy—truly understanding each other before jumping to conclusions. Think of it as a conversation where both work together to build a future, not competing against each other.

The first step is to create a safe space where both partners can openly share their vulnerabilities and dreams without fear. In this space, listening is vital—not just hearing words but also feeling the emotions and understanding their values. Couples can start seeing a way forward that respects both visions through this kind of deep listening.

Compromise plays a big role in this journey. It's about finding creative ways to blend your ideas and aspirations to build something new that neither could achieve alone. In remarriage, where emotions and stakes are high, finding these creative compromises is crucial and shows the strength of the relationship.

The real growth opportunity comes when you face these differences head-on. Each disagreement or challenge is a chance to learn more about each other and yourselves. It's about discovering new things about your desires, strengths, and capacity to love and compromise.

Navigating these differences means always being ready to adapt and grow, ensuring that your relationship doesn't just endure but gets stronger with each challenge. In remarriage, true harmony comes not from avoiding conflict but from embracing it as a part of your shared journey, using it to deepen your understanding and love.

The Role of Rituals in Strengthening Your Bond

The little routines you create together really help strengthen your bond. These rituals might seem small—like having coffee together in the morning or saying goodnight especially—but they turn everyday moments into something meaningful. They provide comfort and a reason to celebrate the ordinary parts of your life together. As days go by, these rituals become the rhythm of your relationship, keeping you connected and close.

Daily Rituals

In the middle of busy schedules and the constant ticking of the clock, finding little moments of peace where you can connect with your partner is key. These daily rituals become small havens of together-ness that keep your relationship solid and in the moment. Think about starting your day by sharing a coffee in the quiet morning, just you two whispering about your hopes or worries. Or taking a walk together in the evening, chatting about anything and everything as the day winds down. These simple acts might not seem like much, but they're influential in keeping you connected day after day.

Rituals of Appreciation

In a relationship, showing gratitude and affection is more than just being polite—it's crucial to strengthening your connection. Simple acts of appreciation, like leaving a note for your partner to find, sending a text to make them smile during a busy day, or just a gentle touch to say "I see you" really make a difference. These gestures let your partner know they're seen, valued, and loved. They turn everyday moments into extraordinary memories filled with gratitude and affection.

Crisis Rituals

If daily rituals of connection and appreciation make your relationship solid and beautiful, then the routines you fall back on in tough times make it resilient. When life throws challenges your way, having certain rituals can act like beacons, guiding you and your partner back to each other and to the safety of your bond. These might be a moment of shared silence that shows you both recognize the seriousness of a situation, a particular phrase that reminds you of hope and togetherness, or a place that feels like a safe haven. These actions acknowledge the struggle but reaffirm your commitment to face it together, offering comfort and drawing strength from the unity that comes from overcoming adversity.

All these rituals—whether daily, appreciative, or for crises—recognize something special in the ordinary, showing how powerful it is to have shared practices that strengthen your bond. They serve as milestones in your relationship's journey, providing a roadmap and a reminder of where you both feel most at home. By intentionally creating and maintaining these rituals, you fill your relationship with continuity, depth, and resilience, turning every day into a shared adventure filled with moments of connection, appreciation, and solid support.

Communication as a Tool for Vision Building

When two people combine their dreams and experiences to create a shared life, good communication is like setting the pace for their journey together. They swap ideas and listen to each other, crafting a future that includes bits of both their lives. In these exchanges, dreams get a voice, differences are understood, and a clear path takes shape.

The real heart of this process beats when both partners sit down to hash out the vision they're trying to turn into reality. These conversations are more than just talking; they're like sacred sessions where they paint the future together, combining their hopes into one shared dream. In these talks, everyone must feel free to dream out loud without fear, treating each idea as a valuable part of the whole picture.

Listening well is crucial here. It's about thoroughly engaging, not just waiting for your turn to speak but trying to understand and see things from your partner's perspective. This kind of deep listening turns simple talks into a discovery journey, blending aspirations and building mutual understanding.

Feedback and the willingness to adapt keep this conversation going and relevant. Giving feedback in a caring and constructive way shows you're committed to the shared future, and being open to receiving it helps the vision stay dynamic and responsive to changes. This isn't about making concessions; it's about growing together, recognizing that change is a part of life and an opportunity to deepen and refine your shared goals.

Communication is like painting a picture together in the grand scheme of things, especially in a remarried life that blends past and present while looking ahead. Through open and meaningful discussions, attentive listening, and flexible feedback, couples create a future that's not just shared but deeply valued. This ongoing process is key to building a life together, filled with spoken and understood words, shared dreams, and a commitment to a future built on mutual love and understanding.

Revisiting and Revising Your Life Vision Together

It's important to review your plans and goals periodically. This isn't just a routine check-in; it's a deep commitment to ensuring you're both on the same page and adapting as things change. These moments of reflection and adjustment show how dedicated you are to each other and the life you're building together. When you do this, you realize that your shared vision isn't just a fixed target—it grows and changes with you.

Annual Reviews: A Time for Celebration and Adjustment

Holding an annual vision review is like setting aside a special time each year to celebrate achievements, recognize challenges, and plan for the future with intention. Think of it as a regular meeting and a meaningful gathering dedicated to reflecting on shared dreams and experiences. During this time, you take a moment to appreciate the big and small accomplishments of the past year, each seen as an important part of your journey together. It's more than just giving each other a pat on the back; it's about truly feeling grateful for how far you've come.

But these reviews are not just about celebration but also about strategically planning what's next. With a clear view of the past year, you and your partner can have a deep, honest conversation about your dreams and how they evolve. This talk is a chance to touch base on goals that may have seemed far off and plant new ideas that can grow in the future. By respecting and understanding each other, this conversation helps you reshape your shared vision, taking lessons from the past and hopes for the future into account.

Adaptation to Life Changes: Strategies for Evolving Together

Change is a given in life, showing up in various ways and often without warning. When sharing a life with someone, your plans must be flexible enough to accommodate these changes. Adapting your shared vision when unexpected things happen allows you to turn challenges into opportunities. The real strength in a relationship comes from being adaptable and not sticking too rigidly to one path.

Adapting might mean tweaking your goals or rethinking what you want. Navigating this involves staying one step ahead, anticipating changes before they happen, and being ready to adjust. Keeping an open line of communication about new challenges and opportunities helps you both stay resilient and view change as something you can manage together rather than something to fear.

When significant life events happen, whether they're happy occasions like adding a new family member or tough times like health issues or job problems, your shared vision acts like a guiding light. Revisiting and adjusting your plans isn't just helpful; it's essential. It helps keep your relationship focused on what you both want to achieve, ensuring that even in times of uncertainty, the core of your shared dream stays alive and well.

Reaffirmation of Commitment: Strengthening the Bonds of Partnership

Revisiting and revising your shared life vision is a profound way of recommitting to each other and the plans you've made together. This process, often during annual reviews or through ongoing adjustments, shows your dedication to your relationship and the life you're building together. Your bond strengthens when you refine your vision based on new challenges or successes.

In this process, you're not just recommitting to your goals but also reinforcing the trust and closeness that is the foundation of your relationship. It's a way of reminding yourselves that the future you're planning isn't just a set path but a reflection of your ongoing love and commitment to each other. This love is resilient, flexible, and grows more profound with time.

Through regular reflection, celebrating your wins, and adjusting your plans as needed, your shared vision becomes more than just an idea. It turns into a dynamic journey that you're both actively shaping. It's about being willing to explore new possibilities, face changes together, and stick by each other's side no matter what comes your way.

Celebrating Achievements and Milestones as a Couple

When you hit milestones or celebrate achievements together, it's like marking the rhythm of your shared life. These big and small moments are more than just points in time; they're reflections of the journey you've taken together, the challenges you've overcome, and the growth you've both experienced. These moments show how strong your union is, filled with joy, recognition, and appreciation for each other. Celebrating these achievements helps to weave gratitude, inspiration, and fresh motivation into your relationship, building a history that shows where you've been and what you aim for in the future.

Recognizing and celebrating individual and joint achievements helps each partner feel seen, appreciated, and celebrated. This recognition highlights the effort, passion, and commitment to reach every goal, whether a big career win, a personal health goal, or a financial target you've hit together. In the light of this celebration, each achievement becomes a building block for your relationship's legacy, strengthening your bond and deepening your connection as you celebrate.

Including and respecting each other's values and traditions helps create a shared culture within your relationship. Negotiating differences helps you discover their richness, building a story that celebrates your history and potential. After celebrating, taking time to reflect allows you both to appreciate the journey, the challenges you've navigated, and the lessons learned and to feel grateful for each other's support and the growth you've seen in yourselves and each other. This reflection is a profound moment of connection where you honor your past and envision your future dreams together.

Celebrating achievements isn't just about marking what you've already done; it's also about setting the stage for future goals. These milestones show you what you can achieve together, lighting up your future goals not as distant dreams but as real, achievable targets. With each achievement recognized, you find new energy and motivation to pursue your dreams. This cycle of achievement, celebration, reflection, and renewed aspiration keeps the dynamics of remarriage exciting and vibrant, making your journey purposeful and joyful.

Ultimately, these milestones and achievements are not just ceremonial; they are the glue that holds you together. They punctuate your time with joy, reflection, and anticipation, rhythmically enriching your relationship. These celebrations honor your shared journey and lay the groundwork for future adventures, creating a life together that's as rich in achievements as the love and support that made those achievements possible. These moments of recognition and celebration are the threads that weave a lasting and fulfilling partnership.

The Ongoing Journey of Shared Growth and Development

When two people come together to start their lives anew, they open up a world of opportunities for growth and mutual enrichment. As they move forward together, they share their dreams and create new ones as a couple. This isn't just about learning from books; it's about learning from each other, from new experiences, and from the conversations that spring from their shared life.

Adopting a mindset that values continuous discovery and curiosity can drive a relationship forward. It's like being explorers with a map, eager to see what's around the next corner. As they learn and grow together, their relationship deepens, and their bond strengthens.

Life naturally brings changes and transitions; each stage has challenges and opportunities. Whether it's the shift from the excitement of a new romance to the comfort of long-term companionship or from a busy household to the quiet of an empty nest, each phase requires them to adapt and reimagine their goals and dreams together. Their shared vision for the future adjusts as they do, reflecting their current realities and aspirations.

Building a legacy together that reaches beyond just the two of them into their family and community is a significant part of their journey. This legacy, shaped by the values they uphold, the traditions they foster, and the impact they make, serves as a beacon for future generations. It's like a garden they tend together—every act of kindness, every loving gesture, every commitment to making the world a better place helps their legacy grow.

As they close this chapter of their life and look ahead, the essence of their journey—marked by continuous learning, gracefully navigating life's changes, and building a meaningful legacy—highlights the depth of their connection and the strength of their partnership. Despite life's inevitable ups and downs, their journey is guided by their love for each other, pushing them to keep growing, adapting, and building something bigger than themselves. Together, they are ready to face whatever comes next, armed with resilience, love, and a commitment to keep growing.

EIGHT

Embracing Change and Strengthening Your Bond

In the busy swirl of daily life, with all its tasks and commitments, keeping a relationship strong can sometimes feel like trying to talk during a loud storm. But in these chaotic times, showing love and commitment becomes even more critical. This part focuses on how to keep a good balance between handling life's demands and nurturing a relationship, especially when you remarry.

Nurturing Your Relationship Amid Life's Hustle

Modern life moves fast and is full of obligations, making it challenging for couples to keep their relationship strong and vibrant. The real challenge isn't about making big romantic gestures. Instead, it's about the little moments that happen every day. It's about finding balance amid the chaos and turning everyday routines into something special by paying attention, setting clear intentions, and prioritizing your relationship.

Prioritizing Your Relationship

With all the endless to-do lists and busy schedules, making your relationship a top priority is critical. Think of it as a guiding principle for acting, making decisions, and spending time. A good example is having coffee together in the quiet of the morning before the day starts. It's a simple act, but it sends a powerful message: putting your relationship first, even just for a few minutes. Making time for these moments helps keep your connection strong despite the daily rush.

Small Gestures

Small acts of love and appreciation are significant in a remarriage. Things like slipping a note into a work bag, cooking a favorite meal after a tough day, or laughing together at an inside joke show affection and care daily. These little things are reminders that love shows itself in quiet, thoughtful actions. Regularly doing these nice things for each other keeps the relationship strong, even when you face challenges.

Work-Life Balance

Finding the right balance between work and home life is like constantly adjusting scales—it's all about knowing when to lean in and when to step back because time counts in relationships. You might set firm boundaries on your work hours, keep family dinners sacred for catching up, or maybe decide on tech-free times so everyone can focus on each other instead of their screens. Something as simple as a Saturday morning walk can become a particular routine, giving you a chance to connect, chat, or just enjoy being together, reminding everyone that the relationship comes first despite the ongoing rush of work and everyday life.

Visual Element: The Relationship Priority Pie Chart

The Relationship Priority Pie Chart is a handy visual tool that helps couples see how they spend their time and energy, specifically focusing on how much they dedicate to their relationship. It's like holding up a mirror to your daily life, helping you check if the relationship is getting as much attention as you want or if you need to make changes to keep it front and center despite everything else.

In a remarriage, you combine your past experiences with your current life and hopes for the future. Keeping the relationship strong despite the daily rush is about staying committed to each other. It means actively choosing to love, prioritize, and care for each other every day. By focusing on the relationship, showing love through small acts, and finding a good balance between work and home life, couples can handle the complexities of remarriage smoothly. This way, the daily grind can bring you closer instead of pulling you apart.

Maintaining Individuality Within the Partnership

Merging lives without losing your identity is crucial. It's about finding the right mix of being together and being yourself. Keeping that individuality alive while building a shared life is critical to a strong and fulfilling relationship. It means recognizing that while you have shared dreams, you have unique traits and interests.

Maintaining your individuality in a remarriage is like caring for a garden with different kinds of flowers. Each flower brings something special to the beauty but needs space and care to thrive. Similarly, having your own space and hobbies is vital. They help each person grow and stay vibrant, keeping the relationship healthy and dynamic.

Personal Space and Hobbies

Having hobbies and interests outside your marriage is important for your fulfillment and self-expression. Whether it's painting, playing sports, or diving into books, these activities are a way to show who you are. They're more than just ways to pass the time; they reflect your personality and what you're passionate about. Supporting your partner in their hobbies shows love and respect for their whole self, not just who they are in the relationship. It's a recognition that for your marriage to be healthy, you need to feel fulfilled and happy as individuals.

Supporting Each Other's Goals

Supporting each other's goals is key in a relationship. Whether offering a listening ear, a few encouraging words, or actively getting involved in what the other is doing, this support helps dreams grow. It's about understanding that even though you're in this together, you have your journeys and goals. Being there for each other strengthens your relationship and boosts the satisfaction and pride you feel from your achievements. This kind of mutual support solidifies the foundation of your marriage.

Healthy Boundaries

Setting and respecting healthy boundaries is crucial for maintaining individuality within a relationship. These boundaries help keep a good balance between being together and having your own space. They show that true love respects each person's need for space to grow, think, and be themselves. Establishing these boundaries means understanding your and your partner's needs and carefully negotiating to respect both. It's about knowing when to come together and when to give each other space, with each boundary helping to build a deeper understanding and connection.

Keeping your individuality within the relationship is important when past experiences and present lives intertwine with future hopes. The union's strength comes not from losing yourselves in each other but from the balance between being together and being yourselves. This balance is supported by pursuing personal hobbies, supporting each other's goals, and setting those important boundaries. It's the foundation for a strong and satisfying marriage, proving that harmony comes not from being the same but from respecting and blending your individualities in a way that works for both.

The Importance of Date Nights and Quality Time

When days can blur together with all the shared responsibilities and personal pursuits, setting aside time for date nights and quality time together isn't just a nice extra—it's crucial. This dedicated time, purposely taken from the busyness of daily life, becomes a key way to keep your connection strong and let the romance and deep bond at the heart of your relationship shine away from all the routine stuff.

Planning Date Nights

Planning date nights amid the hustle and bustle of everyday life takes some creativity and a real commitment. It's about carving out special pockets of time where the focus is on each other. One way to ensure these moments happen is by marking them on your calendar like any important meeting, showing they're a priority. Whether enjoying a simple home-cooked meal by candlelight or trying out a new spot together, the key is to treat these dates as sacred and non-negotiable. Some tips to keep it interesting: take turns planning the dates, keep an element of surprise, and maybe set a theme like laughter, adventure, or relaxation for each date. This way, each date night becomes a special highlight in your life together.

Quality vs. Quantity

Building a stronger relationship over time is more about the quality of time together than the quantity. It's an important shift—realizing that fully engaged, meaningful moments matter more than being around each other while doing separate things. Quality time is all about giving each other your full attention. This means putting away phones, making eye contact, and listening—showing that you're genuinely there in the moment. It's about making even the shortest times together count by ensuring they're full of love and genuine interaction. Every moment together strengthens your bond and fills you both with joy.

New Experiences

Trying new things together really shows how love is always evolving. It says that growing and exploring are things you should do together, not alone. When you're both open to new experiences, it brings a burst of energy and fresh perspectives that keep your relationship exciting. Whether picking up a new hobby where you can laugh at your mistakes and cheer for the small wins or traveling to new places where every new sight and sound is something you discover together, it's all about doing new things together. These adventures, whether big or small, turn into shared stories that you'll look back on with a smile, building a collection of memories that add warmth and color to your relationship.

In this way, the time you spend together isn't just marked by the clock and how deep and meaningful those moments are. Making time for date nights and quality time is crucial—it turns the everyday into something special. Every day can feel like an adventure, and it's a chance to fall in love again whenever you catch each other's eyes. You keep your relationship fresh by planning these date nights, focusing on connecting during that time and daring to try new things together. This ensures that your journey through remarriage isn't just walking the same path together but a joyful dance filled with laughter, love, and endless new things to discover.

Handling External Pressures and Opinions Gracefully

Dealing with external pressures and opinions can make things tricky. It's like being in a crowded room where everyone's watching and commenting on your every move, and those comments can pull at your relationship. Staying strong together in the face of all that noise, keeping your relationship solid and protected from outside judgments, is a real test of your teamwork and resilience.

People might judge or have opinions about your relationship, from family expectations to social norms. These can lead to unwanted opinions that might make you doubt yourself. But despite all this noise, it's crucial to stay connected and support each other based on mutual understanding and respect. The key is to face the world as a team, stay coordinated and not let outside skepticism bring you down.

Your relationship should be a strong, safe place built on your commitment and love. Facing external opinions together helps protect the special connection you've created. This unity comes from supporting and understanding each other rather than being inflexible. It's about staying in sync and showing everyone that, while you respect other people's views, what matters and holds is the bond between the two of you.

Setting Boundaries in Remarriage with Friends, Family and Society

Boundaries are like the rules that protect the private space of your relationship, showing clearly what's open for sharing and what's just for the two of you. Setting these boundaries is like making a map for your friends and family. It shows where they're welcome and where they might be overstepping. It's about kindly but firmly explaining your needs and expectations. These talks might feel tough because you're opening up, but it helps strengthen your relationship. Once these boundaries are in place, they help guide how others interact with you, ensuring that all interactions are based on respect and understanding.

Managing Privacy and Autonomy in Your Remarriage

Deciding what to share and what to keep private is vital in keeping your relationship your own. It's about knowing your boundaries and steering conversations with respect. Being selective isn't about putting up walls; it's about choosing what parts of your relationship you're comfortable showing the world. This careful choice helps protect the most private and vulnerable parts of your relationship from unwanted opinions and judgments. It's about navigating what to reveal and making each share a thoughtful decision, like sharing a delicate part of your love that you trust others will respect.

Gracefully handling outside pressures is crucial. It's a dance that needs balance, togetherness, and a firm commitment to keeping your relationship intact. As you move together, your united front and the love you share buffer against the outside noise. This resilience allows you to face the world confidently and continue writing your own story, untouched by others' judgments. This love story is true to your shared experiences and clear of outside interference.

Fostering a Support Network for Remarried Couples

Navigating remarriage can feel like balancing new hopes and old challenges, which is why having a support network is crucial. It's not just about having people to lean on but finding those who understand because they've been through similar experiences. This network acts like a guiding light, showing you that your journey isn't unique and that others have walked this path before, lighting the way with their experiences and advice.

Finding and connecting with others in the community who have remarried can be a lifeline. These connections are invaluable, Whether through online forums that connect you with people across the globe or local groups that meet in person. Engaging with social media groups focused on remarried life or attending local workshops and events can be great ways to build this network. These communities offer a space to share stories and advice, which can add layers of love, resilience, and hope to your own story.

These networks also provide practical support. They can be a source of encouragement when times get tough and a resource for finding professional help, such as counselors or retreats to strengthen remarried bonds. Whether it's a reassuring message, a phone call, or meeting up for coffee, these small gestures of support can make a big difference.

In this shared space, stories and experiences weave together, creating a strong and understanding community. This network becomes like a chosen family, bonded not by blood but by shared experiences of love's second chances and the deep belief that we can all build lasting legacies despite the challenges. This support is vital in remarriage, showing that no one has to go it alone.

The Role of Forgiveness in Daily Life

Forgiveness is crucial in a remarriage—it keeps the relationship strong and loving. It's about understanding that everyone has flaws and sometimes things go wrong. Forgiveness in a marriage isn't just about saying sorry; it's about letting go of the small and big grudges that can build up.

Forgiving isn't the same as forgetting or saying what happened was okay. It's about moving on and not letting past hurts control your feelings. It's a big step towards peace, recognizing the hurt but not letting it dominate your relationship. This act of forgiveness shows that you know mistakes can't be changed, but they don't have to hold power over your emotional well-being.

Dealing with daily irritations also requires a bit of grace. It's about not sweating the small stuff like a spilled coffee or a forgotten chore and focusing instead on the bigger picture of your relationship. Getting hung up on every minor annoyance can distract you from the deeper, more important parts of being together.

Communication is key in this process. It's the way you share your feelings and work through misunderstandings. This isn't about blaming but sharing and resolving issues, turning pain into a deeper understanding. Through honest and empathetic conversations, forgiveness becomes a journey you both take, helping each other heal and grow closer.

This journey of forgiveness helps you both get back in sync and focus on the love that holds your relationship together. Each time you forgive, you strengthen your bond, building a resilient and compassionate relationship.

Forgiveness is the heart of a strong marriage, rebuilt from past mistakes and ready to face the future together. It's about knowing that by forgiving, you free yourselves from past burdens and allow your love to be the purest expression of your bond, healing and bringing you closer in a beautiful, ongoing process of renewal.

Keeping Love Alive: Romantic Gestures and Appreciation

Mixing past and present to build a shared life and keep the romance alive is crucial. It's about consistently showing love and appreciation, strengthening the connection despite mundane routines, and continuously nurturing the relationship to keep it fresh and vibrant.

Small, genuine gestures matter most. Simple things like a handpicked flower in the sunlight or a thoughtfully made cup of tea can mean a lot. These small acts of kindness and appreciation remind each other of the beauty in everyday life and the depth of your connection.

Adding a bit of surprise and variety to how you show affection can also reinvigorate your relationship. It could be a note tucked into a favorite book, a spontaneous day trip to a cherished place, or turning a routine chore into a fun, shared moment. These surprises keep the excitement alive and show that the romance is still there, sparkling like stars in the night.

Verbal affirmations are powerful, too. Saying "I appreciate you," "I love you," or "Thank you" might sound simple, but these words reinforce your bond. They show that your love is active and acknowledged, not just assumed.

Keeping the flame of romance alive with intentional love, unexpected moments of joy, and clear affirmations is like continuously renewing your vows. It's a daily commitment to nurture and celebrate your love, ensuring it stays vibrant and strong through the everyday and extraordinary moments.

Dealing With Setbacks: Resilience in Remarriage

Like in any part of life, when you marry again, you'll run into rough patches where things might get frayed or tangled. These tough times can seem like they're dimming the brightness of your life together, but they also bring opportunities for growth and resilience. You strengthen your relationship by facing these challenges head-on and working through them. Each time you come out the other side, your partnership is stronger and more complex.

Transforming Obstacles Into Opportunities

Thinking of setbacks as hurdles to jump over can make you miss out on what these challenges offer. Instead, if you see them as chances to strengthen your connection and toughen up your marriage, you can change how you handle these situations. It's about using these moments to grow wiser and more resilient together. This shift in how you see things requires you to look deeper into each problem to find hidden lessons. Whether it's a misunderstanding that shows you both need to clarify your expectations or financial trouble that tests how well you can work together under stress, each challenge has something to teach you about strengthening your marriage. By patiently and openly learning from these issues, you can build a solid foundation for your relationship based on better understanding and shared strength.

The Power of Mutual Support

When things get shaky, and it feels like you're in the dark, the real strength of relying on each other and having a strong support network becomes apparent. Depending on each other isn't about weakness; it's a sign of how strong and resilient your marriage is. It shows that within your partnership, there's a lot of support, empathy, and encouragement ready to help you tackle any challenges. Reaching out and sharing your struggles is crucial to trusting and working with each other.

Connecting with others also going through remarriage can be a huge help. With all their experiences and advice, this group can guide you through tough times. Their support and tips can comfort you and help steer you in the right direction, making things clearer as you move forward.

Anchoring in the Vision of a Shared Future

Holding onto the vision of your future together helps when things get rough. You both have put a lot of thought and care into this vision, which reminds you of what you're working towards when times are tough. Keeping your focus on this goal takes a lot of faith in the strength of your relationship and your journey. In these challenging times, this vision grows into something more; it becomes proof of your resilience, showing that despite the obstacles, you're both committed to a future filled with hope and shared dreams.

Handling setbacks is about overcoming tough times and growing from them. It's like a dance where you must be flexible and strong, open to learning from what's thrown at you, and focused on your shared goals. Setbacks aren't just obstacles; they're opportunities to strengthen your bond, reinforce your marriage, and keep moving forward with even more determination and a positive outlook. You turn these challenges into a stronger, more connected partnership, showcasing your love's powerful and enduring nature.

Planning for the Future: Dreams Beyond Today

Combining past experiences with your current life as you plan for the future involves balancing big dreams and practical plans. It's a complex mix of hopes and dreams where commitment plays a crucial role. This balance helps guide and give purpose as you work toward a future shaped by shared goals and individual projects.

Goal Alignment

When planning a future together, your personal goals must match what you both want together—ensuring that these goals don't pull you apart but help you grow closer as a couple is key. It's all about talking things through, listening to each other's hopes and dreams, and finding common goals you both are excited about. You must be open and willing to dig deep into what you both truly want. This doesn't mean giving up what makes you unique; it's about celebrating those unique parts of each other and finding ways to blend them into a stronger relationship.

Adapting to Change

Life is always changing, and this is especially true when you're remarried. No matter how well you plan or how much you dream about the future, unexpected things can happen. It's important to adjust and adapt without feeling like everything is falling apart. Being flexible isn't about giving up; it's about making smart changes and tweaking your plans as you go along to stay on track toward your shared goals.

This ability to adapt comes from keeping the lines of communication open. You should regularly check in with each other to see if your dreams and goals still align or if they need to be adjusted based on new circumstances or information. This keeps your relationship and your plans vibrant and relevant.

Commitment in this context means being dedicated to your dreams and the process of dreaming together. It's about creating a future that's full of potential while staying realistic and grounded. By planning together and being willing to adapt, you're not just focusing on where you want to end up but also on the journey itself, making sure it's one full of growth, adventure, and love.

A Celebration of Shared Steps

Every step you take together, whether easy or tough, adds to your life. Holding hands and looking ahead, moving forward turns your everyday route into something more meaningful. Overcoming doubts and planting new dreams makes the journey important, not just where you're headed. Recognizing every step as a part of your shared life turns celebrating into more than just marking special occasions; it becomes a way to appreciate the good and the tough times and the different experiences you share along the way.

Crafting a Legacy Beyond Time

The legacy of your relationship, built on resilience and careful attention, extends far into the future, affecting more lives than you might see right now. It comprises all the tough challenges you've faced together and the happy moments you've fully embraced. This legacy serves as a guide for future generations. It shows the power of sticking together and how love can heal, connect, and outlast time. The results of your efforts, like two lives joining together, provide personal fulfillment and inspire others well beyond your immediate circle.

A Reflection of Gratitude

In those quiet moments, as the day ends, you feel deeply grateful when you take the time to think back. You remember all the laughs you've shared, the secrets you've whispered, and those quiet moments of understanding. This gratitude appreciates the imperfect parts, the strength you find in each other's weaknesses, and how special it is to have your lives so closely woven together by choice and constant effort. It's like a quiet thank-you to the world for having each other, learning from the past, enjoying your time now, and looking forward to what's next.

Building a Bright Future Together

As the sun sets, your life together shines, showing off all the experiences you've shared and how much you've grown. It's like a display of everything you've been through and a peek at what's coming next. This showcases the beauty of building a life together after remarriage, highlighting the courage to love again, the strength you've built facing challenges together, and the happiness of being partners through it all.

This journey is more than just living together; it's an adventure you share, deepened by your strong connection, resilience in facing hardships, and the happiness each new day brings. As you continue on this path, it becomes an inspiring part of a bigger story, highlighting the beauty of committing to a future together and the exciting possibilities that await.

Now that you have all the tools you need to create a successful remarriage, it's time to share your newfound insights and show other readers where they can find the same guidance. Leaving your honest opinion of this book on Amazon will help other couples discover where to find the support they need to strengthen their relationships.

Thank you for your help. Successful remarriages are built when we pass on our knowledge—and you're helping me to do just that.

Let's keep the game alive by passing on the torch of knowledge and sparking the passions of future couples. Your role in this journey is crucial, and I am profoundly grateful for your help in making remarriage joyful and attainable for all.

Here's to continuing our exploration, armed with new knowledge and a shared purpose. Thank you for being an essential part of this adventure.

With gratitude,
Taylor Reed

Bibliography

Abrams, Allison. 2023. "Post-Divorce Trauma and PTSD." *Verywell Mind*. January 19. https://www.verywellmind.com/post-divorce-trauma-4583824.

Block, Jocelyn, and Melinda Smith. 2024. "Co-Parenting and Joint Custody Tips for Divorced Parents." *HelpGuide.Org*. Accessed April 7. https://www.helpguide.org/articles/parenting-family/co-parenting-tips-for-divorced-parents.htm.

Conradie, Cassandra. 2023. "The Importance of Maintaining Individuality in a Strong Marriage." *Medium*. April 10. https://medium.com/@cassandraconradie/the-importance-of-maintaining-individuality-in-a-strong-marriage-dc0624180fc5.

Cunningham, Lori. 2021. "Estate Planning for Blended Families: Pitfalls and Solutions." *CunninghamLegal*. March 10. https://www.cunninghamlegal.com/estate-planning-for-blended-families-pitfalls-and-solutions/.

Freed, Meghan. 2023. "10 Ways to Improve Communication in Your Marriage and Strengthen Your Relationship." *Freed Marcroft LLC*. June 12. https://freedmarcroft.com/10-ways-to-improve-communication-in-your-marriage-and-strengthen-your-relationship/.

Harton, Oni. 2023. "Common Legal Struggles for Blended Families." *FindLaw*. July 25. https://www.findlaw.com/estate/planning-an-estate/common-legal-struggles-for-blended-families.html.

Huntington, Charlie, Scott M. Stanley, Brian D. Doss, and Galena K. Rhoades. 2022. "Happy, Healthy and Wedded? How the Transition to Marriage Affects Mental and Physical Health." *Journal of Family Psychology: JFP: Journal of the Division of Family Psychology of the American Psychological Association (Division 43)* 36 (4): 608–17. doi:10.1037/fam0000913.

Institute, Wheatley. 2024. "Date Nights Linked to Stronger Marriages, More Sexual Satisfaction, According to New Study." Accessed April 7. https://www.prnewswire.com/news-releases/date-nights-linked-to-stronger-marriages-more-sexual-satisfaction-according-to-new-study-301742711.html.

Lehmann, Carolin. 2016. "8 Steps To Bonding With Your Stepkids, From Stepparents Who've Been There." *HuffPost*. May 20. https://www.huffpost.com/entry/8-steps-to-bonding-with-your-stepkids-from-stepparents-whove-been-there_n_5727bc74e4b0bc9cb04432b4.

LMFT, Nancy Ryan. 2021. "Premarital Counseling for Second Marriages." *Relationship Therapy Center*. February 18. https://www.therelationshiptherapycenter.com/premarital-counseling-for-second-marriages/.

O'Brien, Sarah. 2021. "Remarrying? These Should Be Your Key Financial

Considerations." *CNBC*. November 3. https://www.cnbc.com/2021/11/03/remar rying-these-should-be-your-key-financial-considerations.html.

Ph.D., Jeremy Sutton. 2021. "Conflict Resolution in Relationships & Couples: 5 Strategies." *PositivePsychology.Com*. November 9. https://positivepsychology.com/ conflict-resolution-relationships/.

Segal, Jeanne, and Lawrence Robinson. 2024. "Blended Family and Step-Parenting Tips - HelpGuide.Org." *HelpGuide.Org*. Accessed April 7. https://www.helpguide. org/articles/parenting-family/step-parenting-blended-families.htm.

Watson, Alexa. 2023. "The Importance of Prenuptial Agreements for Second Marriages -." *Jacobson Family Law*. November 9. https://jacobsonfamilylaw.com/the-impor tance-of-prenuptial-agreements-for-second-marriages/.

"Wealth Planning Tips for Second Marriages." 2019. *RBC Wealth Management*. July 27. https://www.rbcwealthmanagement.com/en-us/insights/wealth-planning-tips-for-second-marriages.

9 798991 348225